The Care and Keeping of Sensitive Skin

The Care and Keeping of Sensitive Skin

A Practical Guide to Holistic Skin Care

LISSA BELL

iUniverse, Inc.
Bloomington

The Care and Keeping of Sensitive Skin
A Practical Guide to Holistic Skin Care

iUniverse books may be ordered through booksellers or by contacting:

iUniverse
1663 Liberty Drive
Bloomington, IN 47403
www.iuniverse.com
1-800-Authors (1-800-288-4677)

ISBN: 978-1-4620-4399-6 (sc)
ISBN: 978-1-4620-4400-9 (hc)
ISBN: 978-1-4620-4401-6 (ebk)

Library of Congress Control Number: 2011913965

Printed in the United States of America

iUniverse rev. date: 04/03/2012

Dedication

This book is dedicated to all of the educators, herbalists and natural beauty gurus who set me on my path, and to all of the authors before me who have inspired me to *seek* my own voice in my writing.

To my children: Audrey Lynn and TJ, who have always been a great source of inspiration.

To my parents: Jim and Helen LoSasso, who instilled in me a deep faith in God and all of His creation.

To my brother, Carl LoSasso, and my sisters: Jolene Frease and Jamie Merlo, for their constant support and encouragement.

Also, to my late mother-in-law, Carol Willsey Bell, who authored 88 books in the field of Genealogy, and taught me through example, that I could do anything I put my mind to.

To Susan Markovitch: for her proofreading skills, and for her undying friendship.

To Carolyn Cruz, the owner of Magnolias on the Green: for her advice and guidance, and all of the wonderful opportunities that she has afforded me.

And, to my husband, my companion, my best friend, and my biggest supporter, Christopher Bell, who made this book possible and is always there for me . . . no matter what.

CONTENTS

Preface

At the age of 16, Lissa Bell found she had Vitiligo, which is hereditary in her family. Because her father and his cousin Anna had Vitiligo, which is characterized by small white patches of skin that often start at the body's extremities, Lissa was familiar with the skin disorder. At that time not much was known about Vitiligo, therefore, nothing could be done for it other than bleaching the pigmented skin in order to create a more uniform appearance. It has now been found that Vitiligo may be associated with autoimmune, genetic, oxidative stress, neural, or viral causes.

Over time, Bell researched and read the limited information she could find about the condition. She had gone to physicians who would ask her what it was. At times, as it spread, it was devastating. People sometimes stared and often made comments or pulled their own hands away in fear when they noticed the spots.

As her skin changed, she found that she had to be much more conscious of the products she used. Bell tried brand after brand of skin care and makeup, hoping she would finally find the magic over-the-counter potion that would make it all better. It never happened.

Eventually, she found that she could not use products that contained synthetics without suffering an adverse reaction. The hardest part was avoiding the sun.

In her early thirties, the younger of her two children developed eczema. People would send her son home thinking he had ringworm, and that he would spread it to other children. The doctor gave him cortisone cream, which made his skin burn and did not help. She wanted, as a mother, to make it all better. So she began researching herbal skin care. She developed an herbal soap for her son and the eczema went away, never to return.

Amazed with the results, Bell began experimenting with herbal products for her own skin. In 2009, she started Lissa's Naturals, a line of skin care products for sensitive skin.

Bell holds a B.A. in professional writing and editing from Youngstown State University in Youngstown, Ohio, where she worked as a freelance writer for 15 years.

In 2010, she earned her managing estheticians license and now provides custom skin care for her clientele. She is a member of Associated Skin Care Professionals (ASCP) and the National Coalition of Estheticians, Manufacturers/Distributors & Associations (NCEA), and is an advocate for the Campaign for Safe Cosmetics, The American Vitiligo Foundation (AVF), and the Breast Cancer Fund.

Introduction

Since the 1960s, there has been a growing concern about the effects of synthetic ingredients on our planet and us. Because of this, truly natural and organic products are growing in popularity because of their purity and cosmetic and medicinal value.

Many times, product names are misleading, and we think we are buying something that is natural or organic because, "Hey look! It says right here . . . Natural, well then, it must be, because I'm sure that is regulated . . . right?" *Wrong*! A label is a marketing tool, and terms such as "fragrance," and "proprietary blend," are often used as a catchall term under which is hidden many nasty chemicals that can build up in your system over time and cause serious problems.

It is important to know how to read product labels. For starters, when you see the word "hypoallergenic," just be aware that it only means that the manufacturer thinks the product is less likely to cause an allergic reaction. "Dermatologist tested," means that a doctor has checked the list of ingredients to see if the product will generally cause allergic reactions. That also goes for "sensitivity tested," and "nonirritating," which mean that you have a slightly less chance of developing an irritation.

Also, be aware that skin care products with at least one organic ingredient used in large quantities can be labeled as organic.

People with sensitive skin are not at the mercy of the skin care industry. No more throwing money away on products that don't work and cause more harm than good. No more feeling of despair when you look into the mirror and see thin, dry, aging skin damaged from the elements and the use of products that are not conducive to sensitive skin.

This book is for estheticians who can use this information to help people with sensitive skin and for people who need answers to questions about how they can treat their own sensitive skin or that of a loved one.

It is not hard to find healthy alternatives. To keep green products safe, do not leave containers open, do not share them, and use applicators instead of fingers.

Many green lip and body balms, body and hair butter, oil-based serums, perfumes (with or without alcohol) bath and body oils, and liquid soap, can have a shelf life of several months to a year.

On the other hand, water based products, including some creams and lotions, must be used within six months.

This is not rocket science. People have been caring for themselves and their bodies with natural, synthetic-free formulations for thousands of years. These plants and natural oils are tried and true. They are there for us to use, not just to make our gardens look beautiful, feed our bellies, or season our food. They are there to beautify, heal, and nurture us.

If your skin misbehaves when you first start your natural skin care routine, pay attention to what it is trying to tell you. This is why it is best to start with just a few basic ingredients, and then gradually add essential oils or herbs for specific needs.

Chapter 1

The Best Herbs for the Treatment of
Sensitive Skin

Aloe vera (*Aloe barbadensis*) First aid plant, medicine plant

Gel or juice

Uses: medical burns, sunburn, cuts, wounds, insect stings, bruises, acne and blemishes, scars, wrinkles, poison ivy, warts, welts, skin ulcers, eczema, shingles, and dandruff (straight from the plant).

Actions: astringent, emollient, anti-fungal, antibacterial, antiseptic, antiviral, anti—inflammatory, immune support, wound and tissue healer, and demulcent.

Constituents: glucomannan, polysaccharide, steroids, organic acids, enzymes, antibiotic, amino acid, saponin, and minerals. It contains **phytochemicals**: acemannan, beta carotene, beta-sitosterol, campesterol, cinnamic acid, coumarin, lignins, p-coumaric acid, and saponins. It contains **nutrients**: amino acids, calcium, folate, iron, magnesium, phosphorus, potassium, zinc, vitamins A, B1, B2, B3, C, and E.

Note: It is possible to develop intolerance if aloe is used in excess.

Caution: DO NOT take internally during pregnancy.

Aloe vera gel (a member of the lily family) has been used for centuries as a folk cure for burns, cuts, and skin problems. It is believed that Cleopatra may have used it as a cleanser.

It contains more than twenty amino acids and carbohydrates and is common in first aid creams, shampoos, and other natural body products.

It is known to restore tissue close to the center of a bad burn by inhibiting the release of thromboxane, which is thought to be directly responsible for cell death and permanent scarring. It speeds healing and stimulates new tissue growth. It can also help to heal cold sores and diaper rash.

There are more than two hundred different species of aloe vera in dry regions around the world. It is known to speed the healing of damaged tissue, counter irritation and inflammation, and deliver a slight numbing effect. It also fights infection.

Taken internally, the juice is known to help lower cholesterol, reduce inflammation from radiation, increase blood vessel generation in lower extremities in people with poor circulation, and soothe stomach irritation. It can also be helpful against infection, varicose veins, skin cancer, and arthritis. It can be used as a laxative and is helpful in the treatment of AIDS as well as skin and digestive disorders.

Combined with whipped egg whites, it makes a good firming mask. As an astringent, it has soothing properties. It contains a polysaccharide that helps skin retain moisture.

Because aloe vera gel penetrates the skin very quickly and reduces inflammation, it is used to treat a wide range of sports injuries, such as sprains, strains, and turf burns. To increase cell-healing time, use aloe gel in the initial ice compress. Soothe more into the injury site two to three times per day.

It also relieves irritation from insect bites and helps restore the skin's natural pH.

Aloe vera is rich in polysaccharides, galactose, plant steroids, enzymes, amino acids, minerals, and natural antibiotics.

Because of its antibacterial and antifungal properties, aloe discourages mold and bacterial contamination.

For athlete's foot, apply aloe and allow gel to dry. Apply powder and put on socks. Tea tree oil can be added to the gel or powder.

For Crohn's disease, drink one-half cup of juice three times a day to help heal the digestive tract.

Allergic reactions are rare. Perform a patch test behind the ear or on the inside of the forearm.

If using a commercial aloe product, be sure it is free of mineral oil, paraffin, alcohol, and coloring.

For a healing and antibacterial gel, add two tablespoons of dried calendula, chamomile, or comfrey to one-half cup of aloe gel. Pour the mixture into a glass jar and steep on a sunny windowsill for two to three weeks. Shake daily. Strain and bottle.

For sunburn relief, mix a drop or two of lavender essential oil to aloe vera juice. Pour into a small spray bottle. Spray on skin as needed.

Apply ice or cold aloe vera gel compress directly to hives to relieve itching, shrink wheals, and block further release of histamines into your skin.

Chilled aloe vera gel can also be applied to soothe razor burn.

For minor burns, run affected area under cold water for ten minutes, and then apply aloe vera gel. Combined with comfrey, aloe will help heal fractures and sports injuries.

Calendula Pot Marigold, English Marigold

Flowers or petals

Actions: antibacterial, anti-inflammatory, antimicrobial and antifungal. It is used as a blood cleanser and wound healer.

Constituents: contains salicylic acid and is rich in beta-carotene, stearin, triterpenoids, flavonoids, and coumarin as well as microelements.

This herb can be applied topically or taken internally for its antiseptic, cleansing, and detoxifying properties.

Applied topically as a lotion, cream, or salve, calendula speeds healing and counters infection.

It is useful for minor burns, sunburn, insect bites and stings, sore and pustular spots, mastitis, cuts and abrasions, inflamed rashes, hemorrhoids and varicose veins, and helps to heal inflammatory problems throughout the digestive tract, including peptic ulcers and gastritis.

Calendula is a healing herb for rough, damaged, and problem skin.

A compress or poultice made of the flowers is excellent first aid for burns, scalds, stings, impetigo, varicose veins, and chilblains. A strong infusion can be used and applied cold to treat conjunctivitis.

Because of its antifungal properties, it can be used to treat thrush and help in the recovery from gastrointestinal infection. It is an excellent remedy for inflamed or ulcerated conditions. It can be used externally as a poultice, or used internally to treat gastritis and gastric or duodenal ulcers.

The sap from the stems can be used to remove warts, corns, and calluses.

It is also the most effective herb for sensitive skin. Because of its healing and soothing properties, it works well in baby oil, baby lotion, and baby powder as well as in creams and lotions.

Use as a salve or ointment for cuts, infected sores, grazes, and wounds. It is excellent for diaper rash.

Calendula-infused gel will calm sunburn. Leave on for twenty minutes and blot off. Use every day for one week.

For sprained or strained muscles, apply a tincture following a cold compress.

Chamomile (*Matricaria recutita*) Also called German Chamomile and Wild Chamomile

Flowering tops and essential oils

Uses: facial masks, steams, eye cream, hair rinses, and shampoos, mildly sedative tea also used as a digestive aid. Often found in facial oils, floral waters, and compresses.

Can be used for acne, allergies, boils, burns, cuts, chilblains, dermatitis, earache, eczema, inflammations, insect bites, rashes, and sensitive skin.

When used as a tea, chamomile can act as a sedative and digestive aid.

It is good for treating indigestion, acidity, travel sickness, cramps, inflamed skin, and poor sleep.

It is current in the British Herbal Pharmacopoeia for the treatment of dyspepsia, nausea, anorexia, vomiting during pregnancy, dysmenorrheal, and specifically flatulent dyspepsia associated with mental stress.

Chamomile is commonly used in pharmaceutical antiseptic ointments and in carminative, antispasmodic, and tonic preparations.

It is also extensively used in cosmetics, soaps, detergents, perfumes, and hair and bath products.

Actions: diaphoretic, restorative and mildly astringent, anti-allergenic, anti-inflammatory, relaxant, and antispasmodic, soothes digestion, heals wounds, and acts as a penetration enhancer.

Constituents: sesquiterpenes such as chamazulene and farnesol, which have antibacterial and anti-inflammatory properties.

The essential oil is rich in terpene alcohol (bisabolol), which is proven anti-inflammatory, antimicrobial, and antioxidant.

Phytochemical and nutrient content: Alpha-bisabolol, apigenin, azulene, borneol, caffeic acid, chlorogenic acid, farnesol, gentisic acid, geraniol, hyperoside, kaempferol, luteolin, p-coumaric acid, perillyl alcohol, quercetin, rutin, salicylic acid, sinapic acid, tannin, umbelliferone. Nutrients: choline, vitamins B1, B3, and C.

Two components of azulene are bisabolol and chamazulene, which are powerful antiseptics.

Chamazulene relieves pain, encourages wound healing, is anti-inflammatory, and antispasmodic. It is known to kill the bacteria, Staphylococcus aureus.

Bisabolol speeds healing of ulcers and can prevent their development. It is also antimicrobial.

Belliferone is antifungal. This and chamazulene have been shown to be effective against thrush. (Candida albicans)

Caution: Should not be used daily for long periods, as this may lead to ragweed allergy. Do not use if ragweed allergy exists. Chamomile should not be taken with sedatives or alcohol. Large doses may cause vomiting.

It is one of the few herbs that can be safely taken by babies, children, and adults for digestive problems.

Chamomile can treat mouth ulcers, stomachaches, and colic. It soothes inflammation and treats gastritis, Crohn's disease, and colitis.

In 2008, it was found that chamomile extract, in the form of oil, accelerates the healing of burn wounds.

Chamomile tea should always be brewed in a pot with a cover, because most of the active ingredients are formed in the steam.

Apply topically as an anti-inflammatory. Use the infusion as a lotion on sore or itchy rashes, grazes, insect bites, and stings.

Apply warm chamomile tea bags to puffy eyes.

As a lotion or poultice, flowers will soothe sore nipples and mastitis.

Chamomile has been used to treat menstrual pains since Roman times. It is highly available and easy to grow, harvest, and preserve.

In baths, chamomile soothes muscle tension and eases anxiety and nervous stress that interferes with digestion. Because it is able to calm spasms of the smooth muscle of the intestine and uterus, it is effective in treating painful menstruation.

It also eases the pain of premenstrual migraines.

When infused with oil and rubbed into the affected area, it can ease pain from rheumatism and gout.

A chamomile compress can be used to treat sciatica, and an ointment containing the essential oil is antiseptic and soothing for itching and eczema.

For nervous tension with cold hands and feet, it can be combined with ginger.

Children from six months or older can drink the infusion to help ease nighttime irritability, stomachaches, and to promote a restful sleep.

Breast-feeding mothers can drink chamomile tea to ease colic and digestive discomfort.

Add a small cup of chamomile tea to the baby's bath to encourage a good night's sleep and rub on gums for relief during teething.

Steam inhalation can clear phlegm and help asthma.

Chamomile-infused olive oil is a good massage oil for cramps.

A patch test should be conducted before using chamomile tinctures, distillates, or essential oils, since they are known to cause contact dermatitis in some people.

Comfrey (*Symphytum officinale*) also known as boneset, knitbone, and bruisewort.

Leaves, flowers, and roots

Uses: an effective skin soother and healer. It is often added to ointments to treat eczema and psoriasis. Effective in healing wounds, stomach ulcers, and bone fractures. Binds tissues and stimulates tissue repair. Apply regularly to damaged tissue such as sprains, bruises, sports injuries, and operation scars to promote regrowth and shorten recovery and repair time.

Comfrey is efficient as an ointment, cream, or poultice of leaves and root, and helps treat varicose veins, slow-healing wounds, and ulcers. Only apply comfrey around the edge of an open wound. Apply with caution during pregnancy. It is excellent in antiaging cream, because of its healing and regenerative properties.

Take baths in comfrey to improve circulation. It also alleviates and heals minor burns.

Actions: a cell proliferant that promotes the growth of connective tissue, bone, and cartilage and is easily absorbed through the skin. It is anti-inflammatory, astringent, demulcent, and healing. Comfrey is also used for its ability to break down red blood cells.

Constituents: mucilage, allantoin (up to 0.8 percent), tannins, resin, essential oils, pyrrolizidine alkaloids, gum, carotene, glycosides, sugars, beta-sitosterol and steroidal saponins, triterpenoids, vitamin B12, protein (up to 35 percent) and zinc.

Caution: Avoid excess use. Do not take comfrey root internally, as it is toxic to the liver. Do not take leaf internally during pregnancy or for more than six weeks at a time. Do not apply to open wounds.

Cypress (*Cupressus sempervirens*)

Tree: leaves, twigs, bark and cones, and essential oil

Uses: appropriate for use in cleansers and toners for normal, combination, oily and sensitive skin. It is also used to help relieve some vascular conditions such as varicose veins.

It is useful in body care for stimulating the circulation and treating water retention.

Cypress is often used in anti-cellulite remedies and is effective for improving overall skin tone.

It can also be used in shampoos and rinses for oily hair.

Actions: anti-inflammatory. Contains vitamin C, potassium, silicon, and sulfur.

Constituents: pinene, camphene, sylvestrene, cymene, and sabinol.

Note: The scent is sweeter and softer than pine, yet similar.

Add to warm bath to stimulate and revive aching muscles after strenuous exercise.

Add a few drops of the essential oil to a body lotion. Apply in a gentle, upward motion to varicose veins two to three nights per week. Do not massage varicose veins.

To shake off the cold, mix four to five drops of cypress oil into a cup of milk and add to a warm bath.

Lavender (Lavandula officinalis)

Flowers, stems, leaves, and essential oil

Uses: used most often to make soap, floral water, powder, sachets, sleep pillows, and bath blends, and makes a lavish skin cream, lotion, or perfume. One of the only oils that can be used "neat" (undiluted).

Actions: Sedative, antiseptic, and heals acne. It relieves sunburn, bee stings, and muscle cramps. The oil can also be used to treat headaches.

The essential oil kills diphtheria and typhoid bacilli, streptococcus, and pneumococcus.

Traditionally, lavender is used to treat chest infections and coughs and colds through an infusion or steam inhalation.

It is good for calming anxiety and tension. It also relaxes spasms of the digestive tract.

A few drops of the essential oil used in massage oil will relax muscles and ease neuralgic and rheumatic pain.

Constituents: volatile oil (up to 1.5 percent, containing linabol, linalyl acetate, lavandulyl acetate, terpineol, cineole, camphor, borneol, pinene, limonene), tannins, coumarins (coumarin, umbelliferone, hemiarin), flavonoids, triterpenoids. Spike lavender (*L. latifolia*) contains an oil rich in cineole and camphor.

Note: Lavender blends well with rose and patchouli essential oils.

Caution: DO NOT use heavily scented lavender products during pregnancy or while breast-feeding.

Use the flowers and leaves to make an infusion for a soothing facial wash for all skin types, especially irritated and acne skin.

Ground, dried flowers can be combined with ground oatmeal and used as a calming, gentle facial scrub, and mask for even the most sensitive skin.

Lavender water has a clean floral fragrance. It is gentle, antiseptic, calming, and healing. It makes an ideal toner for dry skin.

Lavender essential oil can be diluted with rose water or witch hazel to treat acne. It also repels insects and sooths and heals insect bites.

Lemon Balm: (Melissa officinalis)

Leaves

Uses: soothing to sensitive skin, it can be used in bath preparations, face cream, body and shaving lotions. As a tea, it quiets the heart and the overactive mind. It works well when long-term anxiety edges into depression. Because it inhibits thyroid function, it makes a good remedy for overactive thyroid.

As an infusion, it relieves anxiety, tension headaches, and insomnia. It reduces feelings of panic and calms palpitations.

Lemon balm is also safe for children and relieves spasmodic pains and stress-related stomach disorders such as acidity, indigestion, colicky pain, gas, and bloating.

It can be applied to speed the healing of cold sores or dabbed on as an insect repellent.

Actions: the leaf is used as an antidepressant, antispasmodic, insect repellent and relaxant. It also relieves gas and can be used as a topical antiviral and antibacterial. It has antispasmodic activities due to the eugenol content.

The oil has an antihistamine to alleviate problems with allergens and eczema. It can be diluted in carrier oil for this purpose. It also promotes menstruation and eases cramps.

A hot infusion is sweat inducing and useful for treating colds and flu. It is antiviral and effective against mumps, cold sores, and other viruses, because of the polyphenols and tannin. It is best used fresh or freeze-dried, because the volatile oils diminish during the drying process.

Constituents: volatile oil (up to 0.2 percent, comprising citral, citronellal, eugenol acetate, geraniol, and other components), polyphenols, tannin, flavonoids, rosmarinic acid, and triterpenoids.

There are no known cautions.

For anxiety, tension headaches, insomnia, panic, and palpitations, make an infusion and drink two to three times per day.

Leaves are best used fresh. It mixes well with anise seeds, peppermint, bee balm, basil, cardamom pods, fennel seeds, and rosehips.

To treat eczema or psoriasis, fill basin with cold water. Add a few ice cubes to make it cold, and sprinkle four to five drops of lemon balm essential oil onto the surface. Wring out a clean cloth, such as old sheeting or a big cotton handkerchief, into the water and absorb as much of the oil as possible. Apply it to the affected area. Chamomile can also be used.

Patchouli: (Pogostemon)

Leaves and essential oil

Uses: shampoo, face cream, body lotion, deodorant, and perfume.

Actions: antiseptic, aphrodisiac, deodorant, antifungal. Rejuvenates cells and treats acne and eczema.

Constituents: caerulein, stearoptene, patchouli alcohol, and cadinene.

Pine: (Pinus salius)

Needles, sap, and essential oils

Uses: bath herbs and infused oils for stimulating the senses and soothing the skin. Widely used in disinfectants and detergents. It is useful for some scalp oils and as a topical antiseptic for spots and boils. A couple of drops in a bath will stimulate circulation.

As a steam inhalation, it helps to fight infection and is effective against kidney, respiratory, and sinus problems as well as asthma and flu. As a salve or ointment, it is used to treat outer mouth inflammations.

Actions: stimulating, antiseptic, disinfectant, rich in vitamin C.

Constituents: pinene, limonene, Terpenine, phellandrene, sylvestrene, terpineol acetate, cadinene, camphene, dipentene, borneol, cineole, bornyl acetate.

Rose: (*Rosa* spp.) or Rose Otto (*Rosa damascena*)

Petals, hips, flowers, leaves, and essential oil

Uses: petals and essential oil can both be used in baths, lotions, creams, oils, and gentle scrubs. Rose hip seed oil is used in creams and lotions to counteract the effects of aging.

Actions: petals and essential oil are balancing, calming, and mildly astringent, antiseptic, healing, rejuvenating, fragrant, and restore pH levels. Helps revive tired, devitalized skin and eyes.

Constituents: vitamin C (to 1.7 percent), vitamins B, E, and K, Nicotanimide, organic acids, tannin, and pectin.

Rose oil is used to ease severe depression and is an effective treatment for dry, aging, and sensitive skin.

Rose hip seed extract is used to promote tissue regeneration and helps prevent and reduce scarring from cuts and acne. It reduces wrinkles and maintains texture, freshness, and elasticity of the skin.

A rose infusion, or rose water, which is one of the least expensive and most soothing astringents available, can be used for a compress to soothe and refresh tired eyes. Prepare the infusion or heat rose water gently over low heat. Allow to cool completely and submerge a clean, soft cloth in the water. Place over the eyes and leave on for ten minutes. Keep leftover infusion in the refrigerator for up to three days.

Deep red roses are the most potent. Place the fresh petals in a jar and pour boiling water over the top. Once the water changes to a deep red color, strain out the petals. Bottle the water to be used as an effective mouthwash that will cleanse and strengthen gums and mucous membranes.

Or

Make a vinegar extract by covering two and a half ounces of rose petals with one pint of red wine vinegar. Be sure the petals are completely covered. Seal the jar tightly. Leave to macerate for one week and shake daily. Strain out the petals and store the vinegar in a dark glass bottle.

To use: spoon one tablespoon of the vinegar in a small glass of warm water and gargle.

Mix rose water fifty-fifty with vegetable glycerin to make a gentle skin wash or freshener for dry skin.

Rose hydrosol is a very effective and gentle eye makeup remover.

The essential oil known as attar of rose and rose absolute, contains more than three hundred compounds that among other things, have antioxidant and antimicrobial properties.

According to Richard Mabey, author of *The New Age Herbalist*, the essential oil, which comes from damascene, centifolia, and gallica varieties of rose are valued for their ability to ease tension in women, particularly for post-natal depression and stress.

Rose geranium: (*Pelargonium capitatum*), Geranium rosata or scented pelargonium

Leaves and essential oil

Actions: mildly astringent. Rose geranium helps to heal burns, abrasions, ulcers, and acne when combined with lavender. It relieves dry and itchy skin, eczema, and PMS. It is safe for all skin types. It can be used as a nerve tonic and is known to have a stimulatory effect on the adrenal cortex, which stimulates the production of corticosteroid hormones, which suppress the inflammatory response and depress the immune processes.

Constituents: geraniol, linalool, and citronellol.

Note: The aroma is similar to rose and blends well with most other scents. It is safe for both children and pregnant women.

An infused oil of rose geranium can be rubbed all over the body before getting into the bath or shower.

Mixed with castor oil, it will easily disperse in the water. Add one part of infused rose geranium oil to three parts of castor oil.

Bottle in a dark glass container and use one to two tablespoons of the mixture for each bath.

To kill airborne bacteria, place two to three drops each of sage, rose geranium, and lavender essential oils in a plant mister half full of distilled water.

Two or three drops of rose geranium essential oil added to a little base oil can be rubbed into an insect bite or sting to stop stinging and itching.

For quick and uplifting massage oil, blend two drops of rose geranium essential oil with two teaspoons of sweet almond or extra-virgin olive oil.

For severe menstrual cramps, mix three to five drops of the oil with a half ounce of carrier oil (preferably jojoba or apricot kernel oil since they are so readily absorbed into the skin). Apply to abdomen or back or wherever cramping is occurring.

Chapter 2

Skin Care Pantry Essentials

Almond Oil, Sweet

Sweet almond oil is a colorless plant oil made from the seeds of the almond tree, *Prunus dulcis*. It is an important ingredient in moisturizing soaps, creams, and skin treatments and can be used neat for hand and nail massage. It contains vitamins D and E and has antiaging, anti-irritant and anti-imflammatory properties.
*Caution: DO NOT use if nut allergies exist.

Almond Meal

Rich in minerals and vitamins, almond meal makes an exceptionally gentle skin exfoliant.
*Caution: DO NOT use if nut allergies exist.

Arrowroot

This powder is used in powders and hair dyes. It is added to moisturizers as a thickener and acts as a penetration enhancer. It is similar to cornstarch, but has a finer consistency.

Avocado Oil

The oil comes from the flesh of the fruit of the avocado tree, *Persea Americana*. The flesh of the avocado contains nearly 50 percent plant oil and is a good source of vitamin E, magnesium, traces of the B complex vitamins, and lecithin. It contains linoleic acid, which strengthens the membranes surrounding skin cells. It absorbs readily into the skin and is perfect for dry, aged, and undernourished skin. The dark, nutty smelling oil is appropriate for soothing dry, parched skin and is excellent for skin creams.

Baking Soda (*sodium bicarbonate*)

This white powder has a slightly foaming action in water and dissolves easily. It is both deodorizing and cleansing. Because it is lightly abrasive and bleaching, it is an effective ingredient in some toothpaste. It is well suited in bath preparations for soothing irritated skin and can be made into an effective, yet gentle antibacterial facial scrub for acne-prone skin. A paste made of baking soda and water will soothe bee stings and work as an anti-inflammatory.

For desincrustation (to lift dried sebum out of pores without the use of electric current), mix one teaspoon baking soda with one cup distilled water. Mix well and apply to the face.

Beeswax
Derived from honeycombs, this wax polishes and protects the skin. It is used in moisturizers. It is good for chapped skin and can be used as an emulsifier in moisturizing skin creams.

Bee Pollen
Added to face cream and body lotion, bee pollen renews the skin. It is rich in protein, vitamins, calcium, and other minerals.
*Caution: DO NOT use if pollen or ragweed allergies exist.

Borax
This white, powdery, naturally occurring substance consists of alkaline crystals. It is used by the body to keep bones and teeth healthy and strong. It can also be used as a water softener, and a preservative and skin soother as well as an antiseptic. It should not be used on broken skin. Because of its soothing properties, it is used in soaps, shampoos, eye gels, moisturizers, and herbal bath blends.

Brewer's Yeast
A by-product of fermented barley, this food supplement is an excellent source of B vitamins including thiamin, riboflavin, and nicotinic acid. It is used in face masks and hair packs for its deeply nourishing properties.

Calamine Lotion
This lotion is made from the root of the sweet flag plant *acorus calamus*. It contains zinc oxide, with five percent iron oxide added to turn the liquid a pale pink color. It has drying and cooling properties and is good for sore throats and sunburned skin. It is often found in astringents and facial washes.

Castile Soap
Made from a blend of olive, coconut, or jojoba oil, Castile makes a wonderfully gentle base for shampoo, as well as face and body cleansers.

Castor Oil
Derived from the beans of the *Ricinus communis*, this heavy, clear oil softens the skin and is rarely linked with allergic reactions. It helps to seal in moisture and is an ideal base for muscle rub. The oil is rich in ricinoleic, oleic, and linoleic acids and is capable of absorbing UV light and enhancing the penetration of other ingredients. It can also be used in lip balms and other products designed to create a protective barrier between the skin and harsh environmental conditions. It works well as a conditioner as it adds shine to dull hair. It is also helpful in treating brittle nails and extremely dry skin.

Cider Vinegar
This vinegar has low acidity and is similar to the hydrochloric acid produced by the stomach. It is used to correct the acid pH balance in skin fresheners and can be useful when added to the final rinsing water after shampooing.

Coconut Oil
This truly vegetarian oil solidifies at room temperature. It is extracted from the kernels of the coconut, *Cocos nucifera*. Because it does not go rancid easily and has low lathering detergent properties, it is a good natural cleansing agent. It can be used in shampoos and gentle washing liquids and is often found in soaps and body lotions. On its own, it makes a good skin moisturizer and helps to fade age spots and acne scars. It is good to use for treating skin following sun exposure and as an ingredient in massage oils. It has a remarkably long shelf life. When mixed with other oils, it will not solidify again at room temperature.

Cornstarch
A good ingredient for body care products, cornstarch improves absorption, helps to soften the effects of acidic ingredients and to increase viscosity. It has cooling, drying, calming, neutralizing and

smoothing properties and makes a good base for body powder in natural formulas.

Dead Sea Salts
These salts have the same effect as regular sea salts, but they are higher in mineral content.

Distilled Water
It is important to use distilled water (not tap or spring water) whenever a recipe calls for water, because it is free of bacteria, minerals, and chlorine.

Epsom Salts
These crystals are an effective anti-inflammatory. They help to reduce swelling and soften the skin. Use in baths (foot and body) and scrubs.

Evening Primrose Oil
This oil comes from the tiny, dark brown seeds of the evening primrose, *Oenothera biennis*. It contains essential fatty acids such as gamma-linolenic acid (GLA).

Gamma-linoleic acid is an extremely rich omega-6 fatty acid, which may be an effective component in the fight against breast cancer. It is effective for autoimmune disorders, arthritis, and eczema. When taken in capsule form, it can treat hormonal problems such as PMS and menopause symptoms, and helps to control eczema. Used as an astringent, it can relieve skin irritation. Evening primrose oil helps moisturize the skin and treats aging and troubled skin conditions. It works well in moisturizers and creams.

Extra-Virgin Olive Oil
Pressed from the fruits of the *Olea europaea,* olive oil is an essential ingredient in many beauty treatments. Olive oil remains stable when heated to high temperatures and resists rancidity. It is useful, on its own, for treating sunburned and inflamed skin. It is often used as a base for suspending other ingredients and can be used on the hair and skin as an emollient. Extra-virgin olive oil has not been chemically refined. It contains both vitamin E and lecithin.

Fuller's Earth

Has the appearance of powdered clay, and it is mined from reclaimed areas of the seabed. Fuller's, those whose job it was to remove impurities from freshly woven wool, have used it for centuries to extract the natural grease or lanolin from sheep's wool. It is absorbent and works by drawing out dirt and impurities from the skin. A good source of silica and other minerals, this clay helps to maintain the skin's strength and suppleness.

Grapeseed Oil

This light, colorless oil is extracted from the seeds and the fruit of the grape plant, *Vitis vinifera*. It is one of the best plant oils for massage due to its fine texture. It is also used in body lotions and lightweight skin creams. It is especially good for oily skin and can be used in place of sweet almond oil.

Green Tea (*Camellia sinensis*)

Whether used as an infusion or an extract, green tea is rich in antioxidants. It has anti-inflammatory, adaptogenic, anticarcinogenic, and antiseptic properties. It is capable of soothing the skin and works well to help protect the skin from UV radiation-induced damage. The extract works well when added to toners, moisturizers and sunscreens, and is effective in the treatment of acne and rosacea.

Hemp Oil

This light, nourishing oil has anti-inflammatory properties and is rich in vitamin E and omega-3s.

Honey

Made by bees from the sweet nectar in plants and flowers, honey is a mixture of 98 percent sugar and 2 percent enzymes, vitamins, and minerals. It is used for its mild antiseptic properties and assists in the removal of dead skin cells. It is best to use dark or slightly cloudy honey, because it retains the vitamin-enriched pollen that contributes to its nutrient content. Dark honeys retain higher levels of minerals. It is soothing in moisturizers, hand creams, and body lotions. Always do a patch test first.

*Note: Use only local honey (produced within 15 miles of your home). This will help to alleviate symptoms due to pollen allergies.

Jojoba Oil

A pale yellow, naturally occurring liquid wax that is derived from the seeds of the jojoba plant *Simmondsia chinensis*. It is an important ingredient in many scalp and skin lotions and is the only wax that is naturally liquid at room temperature. It is a good natural substitute for petroleum jelly and works well as both a lubricant and hair conditioner. This oil closely matches the skin's own sebum. It is used in facial treatments, especially for oily skin, and is effective when used alone to help reduce the appearance of fine lines and other signs of aging. It has a long shelf life and does not spoil when left open. It works well as a penetration enhancer and has an exceptionally long shelf life.

Lecithin

An essential fatty acid, lecithin is found in egg yolks, soya beans, avocados, and unrefined cooking oils. Lecithin is antioxidant, emollient, and emulsifying. It contains vitamin E, phospholipids, and minerals, and it is used as an emulsifier to blend oil-based and water-based substances with one another. One of the skin's own natural moisturizing factors (NMFs); it is found in the membranes of all of our cells and is a vital component of skin tissue, which helps to keep the complexion strong and healthy. It is a natural emulsifier, holding a liquid in a suspension to prevent separation. It is often added to moisturizers to help lock moisture into the skin. Other NMFs include urea compounds, lactic acid, and glycolic acid.

Oatmeal

Oats are a good source of protein, antioxidants, vitamins, and polyunsaturated fats, which are soothing to the skin. This makes oatmeal a perfect ingredient for treating dry, irritated, and sensitive skin. Porridge oat flakes are used to soften bath water and help restore moisture to the skin; finely ground oatmeal is best used to treat delicate and sensitive skin on the face and neck.

Orris Root (*Iridaceae florentina*)
From the powdered root of the Iris, it is used in perfume making for its fixative properties. It is also useful as a natural powder and dry hair shampoo and can be used as a fixative in potpourri.

Powdered Milk
This is also a soothing and softening agent and can be used as a skin lightener.

Rice Flour
Often used in face and body powders, it has a silky texture and is highly absorbent and drying on the skin. It is a good substitute for talcum powder and cornstarch and has a finer texture than arrowroot powder. It can be scented with a few drops of essential oil to make a luxurious body powder.

Rose Water
A by-product of rose essential oil, it is used to soothe skin, but often has an alcohol base, which can be irritating to sensitive skin. Homemade rose water can be made by using witch hazel instead of alcohol.

Sea Salt
This salt is evaporated from the sea or mined from former seabeds. It is used externally to extract herbal properties or to disperse essential oils. It is both astringent and antibacterial. It also has skin softening properties.

Sesame Oil (*Sesamum orientale*)
This oil comes from sesame seeds, which are a good source of iron, calcium, and protein. It is soothing and has little to no smell, which makes it a good choice for skin care products.

Shea Butter (*Vitallaria paradoxa*)
This creamy, solid oil is less solid, but more emollient than cocoa butter. It is derived from the seeds of the karite tree, *Butyrospermum parkii,* which grows in Africa.

It is used as a moisturizer for dry skin, scars, eczema, psoriasis, stretch marks, and arthritis, and as a base for lip and skin treatments. It provides a natural UV protection of SPF6.

Sugar

Organic sugar can be used as a scrub on the body in areas affected by keratinization.

Sunflower Oil

This oil comes from the head of the sunflower plant. It contains high levels of vitamin E and calcium, and it is often used as a carrier oil for the massage blends and body lotion. It is well suited as a carrier oil for the bath. It is easily absorbed into the skin.

Vegetable Glycerin

A sweet, syrupy substance that mixes well with rose water and witch hazel, vegetable glycerin makes a good skin softener, because it is humectant. It is used to make clear soaps, moisturizers, and shaving creams.

Vitamin E Oil

A natural antioxidant, vitamin E oil is a fat-soluble antioxidant and helps to eradicate free radicals from the skin by retarding oxidation. It helps to heal skin wounds, nourish the skin, and prevent stretch marks. Although it will extend the shelf life of products, it is important to purchase it in small quantities since it becomes rancid quickly.

Wheat Germ Oil (*Triticum* spp.)

Wheat germ oil is made from the germ of the wheat stalk. It is the richest natural source of vitamins A, D, and E. Because it is very rich, it is best to use it as an additive to enrich skin creams and lotions. Its vitamin content makes it useful as a natural preservative. It will prevent cream from becoming rancid. It is used in antiaging formulas since its vitamin E content helps to neutralize the free radicals in the skin, which are responsible for most of the skin's visible signs of premature aging such as loss of skin tone and wrinkles. Only a few drops of this oil are needed for use in skin creams and massage oils.

*Caution: DO NOT use if you have allergies to wheat products.

Witch Hazel (*Hamamelis virginiana*)

One of the most widely used plants in Western medicine; the leaves contain high levels of the tannin, hamamelitannin, which gives it astringent and anti-inflammatory properties. It is used to heal veins and skin. These tannins are useful in binding protein in the skin to form a tight layer, which is resistant to disease. It separates the bacteria that has settled on the skin and protects against irritation. It works well in the treatment of sores, bruises, swelling, hemorrhoids, and postpartum tears of the perineum. It is commonly used in cleansers and toners for oily skin, aftershaves, and topical treatments for insect bites.

*Caution: DO NOT take internally.

Zinc Oxide

This thick white paste is a sunblock, which screens out most all of the sun's harmful rays. It has astringent properties and dries the skin. It can be useful in rash creams, antiperspirants, and shaving creams.

Chapter 3

Infusions, Decoctions, Tinctures,
and Emulsions

Naturally, there is a strong connection between inner and outer health. When everything is working properly on the inside, it will show up on your skin and so it is just as important to treat your skin from the inside as well as from the outside.

Many infusions, decoctions, and tinctures can be taken internally and applied externally and so, this chapter includes basic preparations for a more holistic lifestyle.

Infusion

Measure one teaspoon dried or two teaspoons of the fresh herb into a heat-tolerant container. In a pan or teapot, bring one cup of water to a boil. Pour the water over the herbs. Cover and allow the herbs to steep for 10-15 minutes. Strain and discard the herbs. Use the infusion as an ingredient in preparations, or drink as a tea if the herb is appropriate for internal use.

Decoction

In a pan or teapot, bring water to a boil. Add the measured herbs to the pan and reduce the temperature until the water is gently simmering. Allow the herbs to simmer 15-20 minutes. Strain and use the decoction as an ingredient in preparations, or drink as a tea if the herb is appropriate for internal use.

Tincture

A tincture is prepared through a method called maceration. It is used for the preparation of alcohol, vinegar, or witch hazel tinctures, as well as liniments for topical use.

You will need:
1 clean, 1 pint glass jar with a tight-fitting lid
1 cup chopped fresh herbs or ¼ cup chopped dried herbs
1 pint brandy, vodka, vinegar, or witch hazel (witch hazel and cider vinegar are best for sensitive skin).

Place the herbs in the jar. Pour the liquid over top of the plant material until it reaches the shoulder of the jar. Put the lid on tightly and label the jar with ingredients and date.

Store at room temperature 4-6 weeks. Shake every other day. Keep out of direct light and heat. Strain and place a clean cotton cloth or coffee filter in the bottom of a colander or strainer. Put colander into pan or bowl and slowly pour the liquid and herb material into the colander. Allow it to drain for a minute or two, and then pull the corners of the cloth to form a bundle. Squeeze the bundle until all of the liquid has been removed from the plant material. Discard the plant material into a compost pile.

The strained liquid is the finished tincture. Store in a clean glass jar, tightly closed, and clearly marked.

Tinctures with at least 25 percent alcohol content will keep indefinitely.

Vinegar or Witch Hazel Tincture
Use apple cider vinegar or witch hazel instead of alcohol
Allow to set for 2-6 weeks
Shelf life is one year.

Syrup

Warm one cup of honey in a pan over low heat. Add one to two ounces of traditional tincture and cook 10-15 minutes. Simmer gently. Allow to cool to room temperature. Pour into a glass bottle and label with the expiration date. Syrups will keep for six months. Store in the refrigerator and administer by teaspoonful.

Use:
Horehound and sage for coughs and irritated throats
Echinacea and ginger for colds and flu
St. John's wort, passionflower, and skullcap with peaches as an elixir for nervous system support
Angelica, rosemary, and violet for respiratory support

Medicinal Honey

Heat one-quart wildflower honey over low heat until warmed through. Add one cup chopped fresh herbs or one-fourth cup dried herbs and continue heating 15-20 minutes and pour mixture into a heat-tolerant jar. Close tightly. Leave herbs in honey. Do not drain. Shelf life is eighteen months. Use by teaspoon or tablespoon.

Use:
Lavender for a restful sleep
Ginger for circulation
Monarda to soothe a sore throat
Lemon balm to calm an upset stomach
Chamomile to relieve a headache

Crystallized Herbs

Place herbs in a glass baking pan. Cover with honey. Cover with plastic wrap and allow to sit for 2-3 days at room temperature.

Strain out herbs and place in a single layer on a baking sheet lined with waxed paper. Cover loosely with another piece of waxed paper to protect it from dust and to allow for good air circulation. Pour the excess honey into a jar and use the herbal honey for cooking and sweetening beverages. Allow the herbs to set for one week.

Dust the herbs lightly with sugar. Spread them out in a single layer on a piece of butcher or wax paper and allow to dry 1-2 days. Store in a glass jar until ready to use. Will keep 2-4 weeks at room temperature or for several months in the refrigerator. Eat one or two pieces at a time.

Use:
Borage flowers for skin health or rosemary for circulation.

Infused Oil

Place one-third cup of dried plant material in a jar with enough extra-virgin olive oil to cover the plant material.

Check the jar after several hours to be sure the plant material hasn't absorbed all of the oil. If the oil has been absorbed, add another inch or so of oil. Cover the jar with a clean cotton cloth or a coffee filter and secure with a rubber band or a canning jar ring. Do not cover with a lid yet because the herb will sometimes release a gas and could blow the lid right off the jar. Allow to infuse in a sunny window or on a counter top for about 10 days. Strain and discard in compost pile. Keep the oil in a jar for up to one year.

Use:
Mullein for ear pain
Calendula for smooth skin
St. John's wort for first aid oil
Basil for digestion

Ointment

Warm, but don't boil, one cup of infused oil. In a separate saucepan, heat one-half ounce of beeswax. Pour the wax into the warmed oil. Test consistency by putting a drop of the mixture onto a glass plate. Put the plate in the freezer for 1-2 minutes until the mixture cools completely. Once cooled, it should easily spread onto skin. If too thin, add a little beeswax. If too thick, add a bit more oil. Pour into jars. Cool completely. Cover and label. Shelf life is one year.

Salve

Use the instructions for ointment but increase the amount of beeswax to one ounce.

Use:
Calendula for scrapes, cuts, and abrasions
Lemon balm for cracked lips
Lavender for headaches
Comfrey to prevent scarring
Marshmallow use as an antibacterial and to soothe skin irritation

Emulsion

In the top of a double boiler, combine one cup of infused oil with one-half cup beeswax beads, and stir until beeswax is melted and well combined. Remove from heat and continue stirring. As the mixture cools, it will become creamy. Continue stirring until completely cooled and transfer to a wide-mouthed jar with a tight-fitting lid. Label and date with an expiration date of one or two months. Refrigerating the mixture will extend the shelf life.

Medicinal Butter

Heat one ounce of coconut oil or shea butter over very low heat. Add one-quarter to one-half teaspoon each of powdered herb of choice. Mix well and remove from heat. Allow to cool slightly but not until thickened and pour into mini ice cube trays. Place in freezer until hardened. Remove from tray and place in labeled freezer bag. Store mini-cubes in the freezer until one hour before using. This mixture will keep nicely in the freezer for up to eighteen months. To use, allow one cube to soften at room temperature in a covered container. When softened, apply butter topically to affected area and massage into skin gently.

Chapter 4

Skin Food

Going green isn't as difficult or as expensive as some people would have us believe. Yes, it is important that our bodies get all of the essential vitamins and minerals they need to work at their optimum levels, but those vitamins and minerals don't always need to come in little capsules. They should also be in the food you eat and the products you use on your skin since they are more readily absorbed in their natural form.

Nutrients

Lecithin—Helps rebuild cells.
Found naturally in raw egg yolks and can be purchased in bead or liquid form for use in treatment creams and masks.

Vitamin A—Helps to lubricate and heal the skin.
Found naturally in green and yellow vegetables such as carrots, spinach, pumpkin, cantaloupe, and cod liver oil. A powdered greens supplement can be made into an effective mask when blended with a carrier oil or distilled water. Carrot seed oil can be mixed with a small amount of carrier oil such as jojoba or coconut oil to be used as an effective treatment for the delicate skin around the eyes. Organic canned pumpkin is an effective and gentle exfoliant.
Caution: Too much vitamin A can cause the skin to turn a yellowish color. Pregnant women should not take vitamin A supplements, because excessive levels of vitamin A can cause birth defects.

Vitamin C—Helps heal cuts. This anti-inflammatory is also an excellent treatment for fine lines and wrinkles.
Found naturally in citrus fruits, broccoli, and green peppers.
Lemon essential oil can be used in masks and creams. Lemon juice can also be added to masks and is a good base for a pH balancing spritzer.

Vitamin D—Assists in the absorption of calcium.
Found naturally in fish, milk, cheese, and yogurt. Unfortunately, sensitive skin cannot tolerate excessive sunlight exposure, but it is important to have at least fifteen minutes of sun exposure per day

to help the body manufacture vitamin D. Milk and yogurt are both effective and gentle exfoliants and are wonderful skin soothers and softeners that can be easily added to masks and scrubs. They are also excellent bath additives.

Vitamin E—This antioxidant promotes elasticity of the skin and reduces the appearance of fine lines and wrinkles. It is found naturally in eggs, wheat germ, whole grains, broccoli, leafy greens, and vegetable oils. Liquid vitamin E is easily combined into creams and lotions, and acts as a natural preservative.

Wheat germ and finely ground grains make good exfoliants for the body.

Oils

Carrier oils, which are often used as base oils for aromatherapy massage blends and emulsions are the best choice for pre-cleansing oil.

Sweet almond oil is a rich emollient derived from the kernel of a sweet, ripe almond. It is light in color and virtually odorless, so that it blends well with any essential oil. Although it is usually safe for sensitive skin, it should not be used by those who have nut allergies. The shelf life is moderate.

Apricot kernel oil is much like the skin's own sebum in weight. It is nourishing and easily absorbed so it will not lay on the surface of the skin.

Avocado oil is a good source of vitamin E, magnesium, B complex vitamins, lecithin, and linoleic acid, which strengthens the membranes surrounding skin cells. This is an excellent oil for dry skin, but may cause irritation for some people.

Coconut oil is full of saturated fat and solidifies at room temperature unless it is blended with other oils. It has a very long shelf life and is a wonderful natural cleanser and moisturizer for skin that has been exposed to the sun.

Grapeseed oil is a lightweight, nearly odorless oil that works well as a base for aromatherapy blend massage oils.

Jojoba oil is a liquid wax derived from the jojoba plant, closely matches the skins own sebum, and is easily and quickly absorbed into the skin. It is very nourishing and has a lengthy shelf life.

Olive oil, particularly extra-virgin, has a high resistance to rancidity, and is the only oil that remains stable when heated to high temperatures. Extra-virgin olive oil is not chemically refined. It contains vitamin E and lecithin and has a rich olive scent.

Safflower oil is used frequently as a massage oil, because it is of medium weight and has a long shelf life.

Sesame oil is a good source of iron, calcium, and protein. It is soothing and has little odor.

Sunflower oil is extracted from the seeds of the sunflower plant. It is best to purchase the unrefined oil from a health food store since it is high in vitamin E and calcium content. It works well as a base for bath blends.

Walnut oil contains high levels of vitamin E. It can be used in place of almond oil.

Vegetable oils can be added to any mask, cream, or scrub for added moisturizing and healing properties. They are also useful on their own for pre-cleansing. Often, it is a good idea, even for sensitive skin, to use a pre-cleansing oil on the face and neck area in order to loosen dirt and surface debris prior to cleansing.

As we know, each one of these oils helps us to maintain optimum health by fulfilling our dietary needs. What we are now learning, is that the same nutrients that keep us healthy from the inside out, are just as effective at helping us from the outside in. Our skin is our largest organ, and if we smear it with chemicals and pollutants, they will be absorbed into our bodies, affecting not only our skin, but our internal organs as well. It is important to learn to feed your skin with a nutrient-rich diet. If you care for your skin, it will protect you and help you to live a long and healthy life.

Fruits and Vegetables

Apples are a source of alpha hydroxy acid, which is effective in exfoliants, peels, and masks. The juice contains phenols, which are powerful antioxidants.

Apricots are an effective antioxidant. The oil can be used as a carrier oil and the kernel can be ground to be used as an exfoliant.

Avocados are a good source of potassium and vitamins B, E, and K. The oil can be used as carrier oil or on its own as a rich emollient.

Beets are antioxidant and the rich red color can be used as a stain for both lips and cheeks, or added to cosmetic preparations as a natural dye.

Carrots are antioxidant, help dry skin to produce sebum, and protect the skin from UV-induced damage.

Coconuts are emollient and most often used for their oil, which acts as an effective barrier cream.

Corn is used for its starch, which is a safe alternative to talc.

Cucumbers contain vitamin A, B6, thiamin, folate, pantothenic acid, magnesium, phosphorus, copper, and manganese. They are soothing and helpful in reducing the appearance of dark, under-eye circles due to their mild bleaching properties.

Green tea is rich in antioxidants and catechins. It has both anti-inflammatory and antiseptic properties. It can help to protect

37

the skin from UV exposure. It can be used in the form of an extract or as an additive to toners and skin creams.

Honey is antibacterial, anti-inflammatory, and antibiotic.
*Note: Use only local honey (within 15 miles of your home), when pollen allergies are present.

Lemons are an effective astringent and helpful in lightening dark pigmentation. The juice is antibacterial.

Chapter 5

Face Care Formulary

Many over the counter facial cleansers are filled with harsh surfactants. The word surfactant is a shortened term for "surface-active agent," which stabilizes oil and water mixtures by reducing surface tension between the oil and water molecules, preventing separation.

Many of the same surfactants found in household detergents are also found in skin care and other personal hygiene products.

The most common surfactants used are sodium lauryl sulfate, ammonium lauryl sulfate, TEA (TEA lauryl sulfate), sodium laureth sulfate, ammonium laureth sulfate, and alpha olefin sulfonate. These ingredients are used simply to produce suds.

According to a report by Mastey de Paris, a leading innovator in the beauty industry since the early fifties, there are two types of surfactants: linear alkyl and ethoxylated. These substances are almost identical except that ethoxylated surfactants have been chemically combined with ethylene oxide, which creates sodium laureth sulfate, which creates 1,4-dioxane, a known carcinogen that has been found in many popular baby shampoos and bath products.

This compound, even when used in percentages as low as 2 percent, has the strong potential to irritate the skin. The report further explains that the high risk of irritation is because surfactant molecules remain on the skin even after washing, stripping away fatty acids, moisture, and amino acids. This process disturbs the healthy growth of the skin, contributing to dysfunctional keratinization of skin cells. Beauty professionals are exposed to high levels of these chemicals on a daily basis. They often suffer from dull, dry, chapped, and peeling skin on their hands due to exposure. (http://www.mastey.net/scienceBrowse.php?cp=35)

According to recent studies, the levels of 1,4-dioxane are cumulative, which means they are stored in the body and build up over time.

This compound may also be present in products that contain PEG, polyethylene, polyethylene glycol, polyoxyethylene, polysorbate, or ingredients ending in—eth—or oxynol-.

In February of 2011, the Society for Women's Health Research (SWHR) and the Personal Care Products Council (PCPC), hosted the Science of Cosmetics briefing on Capitol Hill at which Deputy Director of the Cosmetic Ingredient Review (CIR), Halyna Breslawec, PhD, explained the approval process for cosmetics and how ingredients are deemed safe. The review concluded that 1124 ingredients are safe for use, 875 are safe with qualifications, 9 are unsafe, and 51 had insufficient data. To date, 2109 ingredients have been reviewed by the CIR, whose mission is to "thoroughly review and access and the safety of ingredients used in cosmetics in an open, unbiased, and expert manner, and publish the results in open, peer-reviewed literature." (Newswise: "The Make Up of Your Make Up" 2/11/2011 9:00 AM EST)

Because harsh surfactants strip the skin of natural oils, the skin will work harder to produce more sebum. The best alternative for cleansing is a facial cleanser with an olive or coconut oil base, such as liquid Castile soap. A gentle, natural soap will remove any oil residue from pre-cleansing and help to soften your skin.

Facial Cleansers

Quick Custom Castile Cleanser
1/2 cup liquid Castile soap
1/2 cup distilled water
2-5 drops skin appropriate essential oil

Mix well and store in a dark glass bottle with a pump top.

Aloe Vera Cleanser
2 tablespoons aloe vera gel
1/4 cup sweet almond oil
2 tablespoons rose water
20 drops vitamin E oil

Mix well and store in a dark glass bottle with a tight-fitting lid.

Aloe Cleansing Gel
1/4 cup aloe vera gel
2 tablespoons liquid Castile soap
2 tablespoons distilled water
2 drops skin appropriate essential oil

Mix all ingredients in a small bowl and store in a dark glass bottle with a pump top.

Aloe Makeup Remover
1 teaspoon aloe vera gel
1 teaspoon jojoba oil

Mix ingredients. Apply gently to face. Use cotton pads to remove excess.

Aloe Vera Moisturizing Cleanser
1 tablespoon aloe vera gel
1/3 cup extra-virgin olive oil
2 tablespoons shea butter
2 tablespoons coconut oil
1 tablespoon beeswax
2 tablespoons rose water

Mix aloe vera gel into olive oil. Set aside. Melt 2 tablespoons coconut oil and beeswax in double boiler. Stir until melted and combined. Remove from heat and slowly add aloe mixture into shea butter/beeswax mixture, while stirring continuously. Stir in rose water. Whisk until thick and creamy. Pour mixture into jars before completely solidified. Do not cover until completely cooled.

Aloe and Calendula Cleansing Lotion
4 tablespoons jojoba or apricot seed oil
1 tablespoon beeswax
1 tablespoon strong infusion of chamomile or calendula
2 tablespoons aloe gel
1/4 teaspoon borax
10 drops vitamin E oil
2 drops chamomile essential oil

Melt jojoba oil and beeswax in the top of a double boiler over low heat. Warm infusion and aloe vera in another pan and stir in borax until dissolved. Remove pans from heat and slowly pour herbal mixture into wax and oil mixture. Whisk until cool, thick, and smooth. Add vitamin E and essential oil. Blend and bottle. Cap with a tight-fitting lid.

Rose Geranium Liquid Cleanser
1 tablespoon rose water
2 teaspoons baking soda
2 tablespoons aloe vera gel
1 drop rose geranium essential oil

Warm rose water slightly. Add baking soda and stir until dissolved. Mix in gel. Add rose geranium essential oil. Good for dry skin. Use as a regular cleanser.

Calendula Cleansing Oil
2 cups dried calendula
2 cups extra-virgin olive oil
2 tablespoons avocado oil
2 tablespoons apricot kernel oil
15 drops frankincense essential oil

Place calendula in slow cooker or Crock-Pot and cover with olive oil. Place lid on slow cooker and set the temperature to low. Leave to infuse for 12 hours. Turn slow cooker off and leave mixture to infuse for 12 hours. Strain plant matter from oil and add avocado oil, apricot kernel oil, and frankincense essential oil. Store the mixture in a dark bottle with a tight-fitting lid. Massage into skin as a pre-cleanser and follow with a mild, Castile-based facial cleanser. Shelf life is up to one year.

Just Olive Cleansing Oil
2 ounces organic extra-virgin olive oil
1 ampoule of vitamin E
1 drop of essential oil of chamomile

Pour the oil into a stainless steel shaker and add the vitamin E and essential oil. (If you have acne outbreaks, replace the chamomile oil with one drop of tea tree or geranium oil.)
Shake vigorously for 30 seconds. Pour into a pump bottle. Keep in a cool dry location. Vitamin E is an antioxidant and acts as a preservative. This mixture will keep for three months when stored properly.
Recipe from *The Green Beauty Guide,* by Julie Gabriel (p. 153).

Rose Geranium Cleansing Balm
3/8 cup extra-virgin olive oil
1 generous tablespoon beeswax
2-5 drops rose geranium essential oil

Heat the olive oil gently. Add the beeswax and stir until melted. Remove from the heat, stirring continually until the mixture is cooled but not hardened. Add essential oil. Transfer to a dark glass jar.

To use: Apply balm to face and massage into the skin with a gentle, upward motion. Remove with a soft cloth and tepid water. Remove excess with toner.

Jojoba Cleansing Oil
4 tablespoons jojoba oil
5 teaspoons sweet almond oil
5 teaspoons apricot kernel oil
5 drops rose geranium essential oil
2 drops lemon essential oil

Blend all ingredients and pour into a dark glass bottle. Shake well before each use. Warm small amount in hand and massage into skin. Remove with soft, damp cloth.

Jojoba Moisturizing Cleanser
2 tablespoons jojoba oil
2 teaspoons grapeseed oil
1 drop rose geranium essential oil

Mix ingredients and pour into a dark glass bottle. Shake well before each use.

<u>Day in Provence Cleansing Powder</u>
1 teaspoon loose organic green tea
1 teaspoon dried rose petals
1 teaspoon dried calendula (marigold) petals
1 teaspoon dried lavender florets
1 uncoated aspirin tablet
1 ounce white clay (Kaolin)
1 ounce rice bran
3 capsules of vitamin C

Crush green tea, rose petals, calendula petals, and lavender florets in a mortar. Add the aspirin tablet, crush it, and blend it with the plant material. Add the clay and blend thoroughly. Add rice bran. Twist and open the vitamin C capsules and add the contents to the mixture. Transfer to a wide neck glass bottle and shake vigorously so the ingredients form a homogeneous mix. Mix one teaspoon of the mixture with a few drops of water to form a paste. Massage it into the face. Avoid the eye area. This mixture can be left on the face for up to five minutes to alleviate pimples, dullness, and uneven complexion.
Recipe from *The Green Beauty Guide,* by Julie Gabriel (p. 155).

Scrubs

<u>Oatmeal Soothing Cleanser</u>
1/2 cup ground oatmeal
1/2 cup powdered milk

Mix well and store in low, wide-mouthed jar. Mix 2 teaspoons with enough water to form a smooth paste. Massage into face and throat. Rinse well.

Chamomile Facial Scrub
3 tablespoons strong chamomile infusion
2 tablespoons finely ground oatmeal

Mix infusion with oatmeal to make a paste. Allow to soften for five minutes. Gently massage mixture into face. Rinse with tepid water. Pat dry, tone, and moisturize.

Lavender Facial Scrub
1/4 cup ground oatmeal
1/4 cup ground dried lavender buds
1/4 cup almond meal

Blend ingredients and store in low, wide-mouthed jar with a tight-fitting lid. Use one tablespoon per application. Add enough water to make a smooth paste, scrub entire décolleté, neck, and face area. Rinse with tepid water and pat dry.

Gentle Herbal Scrub
1 teaspoon loose organic green tea
1 teaspoon dried rose petals
1 teaspoon dried calendula flowers and petals
1 teaspoon dried lavender buds
1 ounce fuller's earth
1 ounce finely ground oatmeal

Finely grind tea, rose petals, calendula, and lavender buds in a food processor. Add fuller's earth and blend thoroughly. Add powdered oatmeal. Transfer to a wide neck glass bottle and shake vigorously until blended.

Use daily by scooping one teaspoon into a dry hand. Add a few drops of water to form a thick paste and gently massage into face. Avoid eye area. Rinse with tepid water.

Brewer's Yeast and Oatmeal Scrub
1/4 cup brewer's yeast
1/4 cup ground oatmeal
Distilled water

Mix dry ingredients well. Using one tablespoon scrub and approximately one tablespoon of water to form a spreadable paste. Allow to thicken one minute. Massage onto face and throat. Rinse off with tepid water.

Oatmeal and Yogurt Facial Scrub
2 tablespoons oatmeal, finely ground
2 tablespoons plain yogurt
1 tablespoon apricot kernel oil

Place oatmeal in a bowl and gradually mix in yogurt and apricot kernel oil. Leave oatmeal to soften for 5 minutes. Gently massage into neck and face, avoiding eyes. Rinse with tepid water and pat dry. Tone and moisturize.

Oat Milk Scrub
4 tablespoons finely ground oatmeal
4 tablespoons white clay powder
1 tablespoon milk powder

Combine ingredients. Use 1 tablespoon per application. Add enough water to make a smooth paste. Massage into skin. Rinse with tepid water.

Baking Soda Scrub
2 tablespoons baking soda
2 tablespoons brown rice flour
5 drops lemon essential oil

Mix dry ingredients. Add essential oil. Place in a glass jar with an airtight lid. This scrub helps to smooth and lighten the complexion.

<u>Gentle Facial Exfoliant</u>
2 tablespoons powdered milk
1/2 cup ground oatmeal
1 teaspoon cornmeal
Water

Mix dry ingredients and store in a glass jar with an airtight lid. Use about one tablespoon of mixture per treatment and add enough water to make a thin paste. This mixture softens and soothes sensitive and dry skin. Recipe from *The Herbal Body Book: A Natural Approach to Healthier Hair, Skin, and Nails,* by Stephanie Tourles (p.35).

Toners

Should I use a toner? Almost everyone asks that question. The answer is, "Yes."

Using a toner is just as important in your everyday skin care routine as washing and moisturizing. Toning restores the skin's pH balance, removes residue from cleansing and helps to draw emollients into the skin.

The key is to use a non-drying toner, preferably alcohol free. Good natural toners include ingredients such as witch hazel, rose water, apple cider vinegar and aloe vera gel or juice. These natural ingredients will help to balance the skin's natural pH without drying it out.

Often, over-drying with alcohol-based products can cause an increase in oil production, because the skin is over compensating for the loss of moisture. This can lead to breakouts and clogged pores. A good toner will calm, sooth, and restore the skin's natural pH balance.

Aloe and Cucumber Refreshing Gel
1 tablespoon aloe vera gel
1 inch chunk cucumber
1/4 teaspoon cornstarch
1 tablespoon witch hazel
10 drops vitamin E oil

Blend the aloe vera gel and cucumber together in a food processor until smooth. Heat the mixture in a double boiler until almost boiling. Add the cornstarch and mix until dissolved. Allow to cool slightly and add witch hazel and vitamin E oil. Store in a jar in the refrigerator. Dab around eyes on orbital bone.
Shelf life: two weeks

Soothing Spray Gel
1/2 cup freshly steeped organic green tea
1 cup freshly steeped chamomile tea
2 tablespoons aloe vera gel

Blend ingredients in a spray bottle. Shake well before each use. Store in the refrigerator.

Lavender Aloe Relief
1 tablespoon aloe vera gel
5 drops lavender essential oil

Pour into a dark bottle and shake well before each use.

Tincture of Calendula
1 1/2 ounce dried calendula flowers
3 1/2 ounce witch hazel extract

Reduce flowers to a powder and place in a wide-mouthed jar. Pour witch hazel over top. Seal and store in a dark location for 3 weeks. Shake daily. Strain and bottle. This mixture will keep for 1-3 years. Note: Use for burns, toothaches, cuts, grazes, and boils

Chamomile Moisturizing Toner

4 ounces distilled water infused with calendula
2 drops carrot seed oil
1 drop rose geranium essential oil
1 drop chamomile essential oil

Pour water into a glass bottle. Add essential oils. Shake vigorously prior to each use.

Astringent Toner for Oily or Problem Skin

1 cup witch hazel
4 drops tea tree oil
1/2 cup chamomile infusion

Blend ingredients well and pour into small dark bottles. Seal tightly.

Cucumber and Elderflower Toner

1 cup cucumber, sliced
3 tablespoons dried elderflowers or 3 fresh heads
1/2 cup boiling water
1/3 cup witch hazel

Place cucumber in a saucepan. Set on low heat. Simmer until soft. Allow to cool and strain. In another pan, add elderflowers and water, heat gently and simmer. Strain. Add witch hazel and infusion to cucumber juice. Pour mixture into a bottle and store in the refrigerator. Use within two weeks.

Lavender Water

2 tablespoons fresh lavender buds
1 cup distilled water
1 cup witch hazel

Place lavender buds in small saucepan and cover with distilled water. Set to medium heat. Bring to a slow boil. Remove from heat. Cover and allow to steep for 10-15 minutes for a strong infusion. Strain and add witch hazel. Pour into a dark glass bottle and keep in a cool, dry location.

Lavender Skin Tonic
1/2 cup lavender flowers
3 cups rose water

Put lavender flowers in the bottom of a screw-top jar. Add the rosewater. Shake well and place in refrigerator. Allow the lavender to infuse for 2 weeks and shake once daily. Strain liquid and pour into dark bottles. Apply with cotton pad to remove last traces of cleanser. Make fresh every few weeks.

Lavender Skin Freshener
1 drop lavender essential oil
1 tablespoon witch hazel extract
2 tablespoons distilled water
1 tablespoon rose water

Combine witch hazel, distilled water and essential oil. Mix well. Add rose water and pour into a dark glass bottle. Shake well. Apply with cotton. Use moderately on dry skin.

Rose and Aloe Toner for Dry Skin
1/2 cup witch hazel
1/2 cup water
4 tablespoons aloe vera gel
4 tablespoons rose water
4 tablespoons glycerin

Pour ingredients into a glass jar and shake well to mix. Transfer to dark glass bottles and store in a cool, dark location. The toner will keep for 8-9 months.

Rose Water and Lemon Toner
3 tablespoons rose water
2 tablespoons fresh squeezed lemon juice, strained
2 tablespoons distilled water
2 teaspoons witch hazel extract
2 drops rose geranium oil

Pour ingredients into a dark glass bottle, cap, and shake to mix. Store the toner in a dark bottle in a cool dark cupboard. The mixture should keep one to two weeks.

Rose Water and Witch Hazel Toner
3 ounces witch hazel
2 ounces rose water
1 teaspoon calendula tincture
2 drops rose geranium essential oil

Blend ingredients, bottle, and store in the refrigerator. Apply with cotton pads.

Moisturizers

No matter what kind of skin care routine one follows, moisturizing is the all-important final step in the process. Contrary to popular belief, a moisturizer does not have to be a thick, heavy cream. With natural skin care, especially for sensitive skin, it is important to stay as close to the natural source as possible. Many moisturizing ingredients work incredibly well in their natural state without having to mix a thing.

It is a good idea to test several different oils in order to recognize clearly their unique benefits.

The ultimate thick, luxurious cream straight from nature is shea butter. Shea keeps its consistency and easily blends with other oils. Coconut oil comes in a close second but can sometimes be a bit frustrating since it does not transport well. This oil melts on touch and does not solidify once it is mixed with other oils. Although, in its natural state, it keeps well in the cupboard and has a long shelf life. Coconut oil is a wonderful base for any kind of skin balm.

Basic Lotion
3 tablespoons sweet almond oil
1 tablespoon aloe vera gel
1 tablespoon beeswax

Mix oil and gel in the top of a double boiler set at low heat. Add the beeswax and stir until melted. Remove from heat and whisk until cool and creamy. Do not cover until completely cooled.

Face Cream
2 tablespoons rose water
2 tablespoons apricot kernel oil
1 tablespoon beeswax
2 tablespoons aloe vera gel

Mix rose water and apricot kernel oil thoroughly in the top of a double boiler over low heat. Add beeswax and heat until melted. Remove from heat. Stir until cooled and thickened. If the mixture is too thin, add a little more beeswax. If it is too thick, add a little more rose water. Add aloe vera gel a little at a time and mix well. Pour into dark glass jars. Do not cap until completely cooled. Use as a moisturizer in the morning and evening after cleansing and toning.

Tea Tree Healing Oil
1 teaspoon apricot kernel oil
10 drops tea tree oil
3 drops chamomile essential oil
2 drops rose geranium oil

Combine ingredients in a dark glass bottle and shake well before each use. Use twice daily on acne-affected areas.

Soothing Face Oil
1 tablespoon organic rosehip seed oil
1 tablespoon calendula infused extra-virgin olive oil
1 tablespoon organic aloe vera gel

Combine oils and aloe vera gel in a dark glass jar and shake vigorously before each use. Store this mixture in a cool, dry location.
This mixture is from *The Green Beauty Guide*, by Julie Gabriel, (p. 195).

Chamomile Neck Cream
1/2 ounce beeswax
2 ounces coconut oil
3 tablespoons chamomile infused almond oil

Place beeswax and coconut oil in the top of a double boiler on low heat. Stir until wax is melted and oils are combined. Remove from the heat. Add chamomile infused almond oil and stir until blended and cooled. Transfer to a jar with a tight-fitting lid.

Cucumber Moisturizer
4-inch piece of cucumber
1/3 cup rose water
3 tablespoons glycerin

Finely chop or blend cucumber and press in a sieve to extract all of the juice. Place the juice, rose water and glycerin into a sterilized jar. Cover and shake well. Store in the refrigerator and use within one week.

Aloe and Lavender Gel
1/2 cup aloe vera gel
5 drops lavender essential oil

Pour gel into dark glass bottle. Add essential oil and shake well to mix. Shake before each use.

Masks

There are several types of facial masks. A remineralizing mask cleanses, draws out toxins, and stimulates circulation with mud, clay, algae, or seaweed. For sensitive skin, it is best to use white clay or kelp. An invigorating mask stimulates, boosts circulation, and re-textures the skin with ingredients such as coffee, seaweed, and fruit extracts. Although coffee may be appropriate on lower extremities, it should not be used on the face or décolleté of anyone with truly sensitive skin. A soothing mask cools the skin with aloe, oatmeal, and herbal blends. Essential oils should be used sparingly.

Aloe Whitening Mask
1/2 cucumber (organic), peeled and sliced
2 tablespoons plain aloe vera juice
1/2 teaspoon milk powder
1/2 teaspoon honey

Blend cucumber in blender or food processor. Add aloe, milk, and honey. Apply to clean, dry face and leave on for 15 minutes or until dry. Remove with a soft cloth and tepid water.

Oatmeal Mask
1 tablespoon ground oatmeal
Rose water

Add rose water to the oatmeal, one teaspoon at a time, until it makes a smooth paste that can be easily spread on the face. Leave on until it dries. Rinse off with tepid water. Pat skin dry.

Oatmeal Herbal Face Treatment
1 tablespoon ground oatmeal
3 tablespoons dried chamomile
2/3 cup boiling water

Pour boiling water over dried chamomile herb. Allow to steep covered for 15 minutes. Strain and discard the herb. Let cool to room temperature. Add enough infusion to oatmeal to make a consistency that will spread easily. Save remaining infusion. Smooth mask on face and leave on for 20 minutes. Rinse off with tepid water. Pat face dry. Use reserved liquid as a facial lotion after drying face.

Cucumber Sensitive Skin Mask
1 tablespoon brewer's yeast
1 tablespoon finely ground oatmeal
1 3-inch chunk cucumber
2 tablespoons plain yogurt
1 teaspoon honey
1 drop rose geranium essential oil

Mix yeast and oats in a small bowl and set aside. Peel cucumber and liquefy in a food processor. Add yogurt and honey and process again for a few seconds to mix. Add yeast mixture to cucumber mixture. Add essential oil and process again until smooth. Apply to clean skin. Leave on 20-30 minutes. Remove with a soft cloth and tepid water. Follow with a light spritz of rose water. The preparation will last for three days in the refrigerator. Recipe from, *The Ultimate Natural Beauty Book,* by Josephine Fairley, (p. 38).

"Peaches and Cream" Glow Mask
1/2 very ripe small peach (peeled)
1 tablespoon heavy cream

Mash the peach half and combine with cream until smooth. Apply mixture to face and neck and leave on for 30 minutes.
Recipe from, *The Herbal Body Book: A Natural Approach to Healthier Hair, Skin, and Nails,* by Stephanie Tourles (p. 64).

Oatmeal Mask
4 teaspoons ground oatmeal
4 teaspoons dried milk powder
Enough water to make a paste

Combine ingredients and allow mixture to thicken for a few minutes. Spread onto face, throat, and chest area. Relax until dry. Rinse with tepid water.

Oatmeal Facial Mask
1/2 cup boiling water
1 teaspoon dried yarrow
1 tablespoon oatmeal
1 tablespoon almond meal

Pour boiling water over yarrow. Steep 15 minutes. Strain. In a separate bowl, mix together oatmeal and almond meal. Add enough yarrow infusion to make a thick paste. Refrigerate leftover infusion to use as a splasher. Spread paste on clean face. Avoid eyes and mouth. After twenty minutes, wash face with soft cloth and tepid water.

Get-the-Red-Out Facial Mask
1/4 cup plain whole yogurt or sour cream
2 tablespoons honey

Stir the yogurt and honey together until smooth. To use, after cleansing, spread the entire mixture on your face and neck, avoiding the delicate areas around your eyes and mouth. Leave it on for fifteen minutes, then rinse well with warm water and pat your skin dry.
Recipe from, *Ecobeauty: Scrubs, Rubs, Masks, and Bath Bombs for You and Your Friends,* by Lauren Cox with Janice Cox (p.27).

Peel-off Sensitive Skin Mask
1/4 cup apple juice
1/4 cup pure rose water
1 packet unflavored gelatin

Mix fruit juice and rose water. Place in top of double boiler. Add gelatin, stirring to dissolve completely. Gently heat the mixture for 1 minute, stirring constantly. Remove from heat and refrigerate for 30 minutes. Spread thin layer over face and allow to dry. Peel off and rinse with tepid water. Pat dry.
Recipe inspired by *The Herbal Home Spa: Naturally Refreshing Wraps, Rubs, Lotions, Masks, Oils, and Scrubs,* by Greta Breedlove (p.95).

Chapter 6

Body Alchemy

Bath and Beyond

During the last forty years or so, taking a bath has gone out of fashion because an increasing number of young girls and women experience reoccurring bladder and kidney infections after bathing in bubble baths and other bath products that contain high amounts of synthetic ingredients. The biggest offender is fragrance.

Appropriate herbal bath blends will not cause skin, kidney, or bladder irritation, and there are many great soothing additives such as ground oatmeal and powdered milk that will leave your skin feeling baby soft. Add a couple drops of sensitive skin appropriate essential oils and soon you will be drifting away into bath-time bliss.

Bathing is not only cleansing to the body, but also to the mind and soul. It is a soothing experience on every level.

Life has gotten so busy that we have forgotten how to take the time to take care of ourselves.

These recipes will not cause harmful side effects; they will relax and renew you. After a rough day, there is nothing like a long soak in a tub to ease your mind and soothe your muscles and aching feet.

Take back the bath!

Anti-Bacterial Liquid Soap
2 ounces grated Castile soap
3/4 cups distilled water
2 tablespoons aloe vera gel
5 drops tea tree oil
15 drops lavender essential oil
2 drops chamomile essential oil

Melt soap in double boiler over low heat, stirring occasionally. Remove from heat. Cool slightly. Add aloe when soap has cooled to lukewarm. Mix oils and stir into mixture. Pour into pump bottle.

Soothing Milk Bath
1 cup milk powder
5 drops chamomile essential oil
2 drops rose geranium oil

Mix essential oils with milk powder and blend well. Dissolve two to three tablespoons in a warm bath. Soak in bath for 10 minutes.

Oatmeal Bath Pouch
2 cups finely ground oatmeal
2 cups whole milk powder
1/2 cup dried lavender blossoms, finely ground
1/2 cup dried calendula flowers, finely ground
1/2 cup dried chamomile flowers, finely ground

Mix well. Divide mixture among 20 muslin pouches and tie with ribbon or string.

Wet Wipes
1/4 cup distilled water
1/4 cup vegetable glycerin
5 drops lavender essential oil
2 drops tea tree essential oil

Mix well. Fold 10 flannel cloths or thick, absorbent paper towels. Place in an oblong, airtight container and pour the mixture over top. Use for hands and face or as baby wipes.

Sleepy-Time Bath Salts
2 cups Epsom salts
1/4 cup sea salt
1/4 cup borax
1/4 cup baking soda
2 tablespoons dried lavender spikes, finely ground
2 tablespoons dried chamomile flowers, finely ground
2 tablespoons dried hop flowers, finely ground
2 tablespoons dried rose petals, finely ground

Mix ingredients and set overnight in a sealed container. Place 1/4 cup in a muslin bath bag and hang from faucet under running bath water.

Relaxation Bath Bag
1/2 cup fresh or 1/4 cup dried lemon balm, finely ground
1/2 cup fresh or 1/4 cup dried German chamomile flowers, finely ground

Mix ingredients and fill each bag with 2 tablespoons of mixture.

Liquid Shower Soap
1 cup Castile soap (grated)
1 cup distilled water
3 tablespoons vegetable glycerin
3-5 drops chamomile essential oil

Mix all ingredients, except essential oil. Warm ingredients in the top of a double boiler over low heat. Stir until the soap is melted. Allow to cool completely and pour into a dark glass bottle with a pump top.

Bath Vinegar
1 cup cider or wine vinegar
1 tablespoon borax
1 teaspoon vanilla extract
4 tablespoons rose petals
1/4 cup rose water
1/4 cup witch hazel

Place first five ingredients in a glass jar with a lid. Shake well to blend. Allow to steep in a warm location for two weeks. Strain through a coffee filter. Add rose water and witch hazel. Pour into dark glass bottle. Shake well. Store the vinegar in a cool, dry location.
To use: add 1/4 to 1/2 cup to bath.

Comfrey Infusion Bath
2 tablespoons fresh comfrey or 1 tablespoon dried
2 cups boiling water

Place comfrey in a 1-pint jar. Pour boiling water over top and steep, covered, for 20 minutes.
To use: add infusion to bath (half full). Relax in the tub for 10-20 minutes.

Green Tea Bath Salts
1 cup grapeseed oil
1 tablespoon baking soda
1/2 cup Epsom salts
1 drop lavender essential oil
1 drop frankincense essential oil
1/2 cup green tea infusion

Mix first five ingredients and store in a jar with a tight-fitting lid. Add a half cup of the infusion to running bath water. Add salts just before getting in.

Winter Soothing Bath Blend
1/4 cup dried chamomile flowers
1 cup dried lavender buds
1 cup powdered oatmeal
1 cup dried rose petals

Put 2-4 tablespoons of mixture into small unbleached muslin bag and tie with a ribbon or string. Tie the bag onto the spigot or showerhead so water can run through the bag. When done, let the bag dry and discard the contents. Rinse the bag thoroughly, dry, and re-use for next bath.

Balancing Lavender Soak
3 cups dried lavender flowers
2 cups oatmeal
1/2 cup baking soda
1/3 cup sea salt

Blend all ingredients in a food processor until finely ground. Transfer to jar and seal tightly. To use: Pour 1/2 cup under running bath water or place in a bath bag to use as a wash bag or tub tea.

Lavender Oatmeal Bath
1/3 cup oatmeal, finely ground
1 tablespoon dried lavender buds, finely ground

Mix oatmeal with lavender. Place in a bath bag. Attach to faucet or showerhead, under running water. If using for a bath, allow the bag to soak directly in the tub for a few minutes before bathing and use it as a wash bag.

Oatmeal Bath Bag
1/2 cup oatmeal
1/2 cup powdered milk
4 tablespoons almond meal
16 drops essential oil

Mix dry ingredients and add essential oil. Place mixture in a glass jar with a tight-fitting lid. Put 2-4 tablespoons in a muslin bath bag. Hang from faucet under running bath water.

Soothing Bath Blend
1 cup dead sea salt
1 cup cornmeal
1 cup dried rose petals, finely ground
1/2 cup dried hops flowers, finely ground
1/2 cup dried chamomile flowers, finely ground
1/2 cup dried calendula flowers, finely ground

Add 1/4-1/2 cup of mixture to running bath water or place 1/4 cup of mixture into bath bag for a tub tea or a wash bag.

Apricot Body Scrub
1/4 cup fine sea salt
1/4 cup apricot kernel oil
15-20 drops essential oil (optional)

Mix all ingredients and store in a low wide-mouthed jar.

Oaty Goodness
1 3/4 oz. finely ground oatmeal
1 3/4 oz. grated pure Castile soap
1 3/4 oz dried, finely ground lavender buds

Combine ingredients and place one to two tablespoons in muslin bath bag or in the center of a small piece of muslin and tie closed. Soak the bag under warm water until the soap flakes become soft. Use the bag like a bar of soap.
Recipe from *The Holistic Beauty Book,* by Star Khechara, (p. 89).

Herbal Body Spritzer
1/4 cup rose water
1/4 cup lavender water
1/4 cup chamomile water

Pour contents into a dark glass bottle. Seal tightly and shake well before each use. Will keep one week. Use after bath as a spritzer or straight out of the fridge to cool down on hot days. Can also be used as a toner.

Lavender Water
2 tablespoons lavender flowers
3 tablespoons distilled water
1 teaspoon witch hazel
2 drops lavender essential oil

Leave to infuse in a bottle for 1 week. Strain and use liquid as light perfume, after-bath splash, or light deodorant.

Lavender-Mint Foot Spritzer
3 tablespoons dried lavender buds
2/3 cups distilled water
5 tablespoons vegetable glycerin
5 tablespoons witch hazel
6 drops peppermint essential oil

Place dried lavender in small saucepan and cover with distilled water. Bring to a slow boil. Cover and infuse for 15 minutes. Strain and discard plant matter. Allow to cool. Mix in glycerin, witch hazel, and essential oil. Store in spritzer bottle. Keep refrigerated.

Calendula Eye Soother
2 tablespoons dried calendula flowers
1/3 cup distilled water

Place blossoms in a pan of water and bring to a boil. Reduce heat. Cover and simmer for 10 minutes. Strain and allow the infusion to cool to room temperature. Soak cotton pads in solution and squeeze out excess liquid. Place over the eyes. Leave on for 15 minutes. Remove and discard. Store the leftover infusion in the refrigerator for up to three days.
Note: Can also be used as a skin tonic or a rinse for fair hair.

Soothing Oil
3 teaspoons jojoba oil
2 drops chamomile essential oil

Shake well. Pour into small dark bottle and store in cool, dark cabinet. Add to bath or use for massage.

Instant Anti-cellulite Oil
1 fluid ounce apricot kernel oil
10 drops cypress essential oil

This can be used as a massage oil or add 8 drops to bath water.

Chamomile and Calendula Oil
1 1/4 ounce dried chamomile flowers
1 1/4 ounce dried calendula flowers, chopped
10 fluid ounces sweet almond oil
1 fluid ounce wheat germ oil

Place dried plant matter in slow cooker. Add almond oil. Cover and set on low. Allow to infuse for 12 hours. Keep covered and turn slow cooker off. Allow mixture to infuse for 12 more hours. Strain and discard plant matter. Place in dark bottle with tight-fitting lid.

Calendula Oil
2 cups dried calendula flowers
1 quart extra-virgin olive oil

Pour olive oil into a slow cooker and set to low. Add flowers. Stir to coat petals. Cover and allow to infuse for 12 hours. Keep the mixture covered and turn slow cooker off. Allow the mixture to infuse for 12 more hours. Strain and discard the plant matter. Add vitamin E oil to the infused oil. Store in the refrigerator and use within six months.

Lavender Body Oil
1 teaspoon avocado oil
1 teaspoon apricot kernel oil
1/4 teaspoon rosehip seed oil
1/4 teaspoon wheat germ oil
1/4 teaspoon castor oil
4 drops lavender essential oil

Blend ingredients in dark glass bottle. Shake well before each use.

Lavender Hand and Body Lotion
1/2 cup distilled water
2 teaspoons dried lavender buds
1/4 cup almond oil
1/4 cup safflower oil
1/4 teaspoon borax
1 teaspoon beeswax
10 drops lavender essential oil

Make the infusion by pouring boiling distilled water over lavender buds. Cover and allow to steep 15-20 minutes. Strain and discard plant matter. Add borax and stir until dissolved. In another pan, heat almond and safflower oil together on low heat, or in the top of a double boiler, set on low. Add beeswax and stir until melted. Remove from heat. Pour infusion into oil and beeswax mixture, stirring constantly. Stir until cool. Store the cream in dark glass, pump-top bottles.

Body Butter
4 ounces shea butter
2 fluid ounces apricot kernel oil
20 drops rose geranium essential oil

Place shea butter and apricot kernel oil in food processor and blend until creamy. Add essential oil and blend. Transfer to jar. Shelf life is six months.

All-Purpose Calendula Skin Salve
1 1/2 cup dried calendula flowers
5/8 cup apricot kernel oil
1/4 cup beeswax

Place calendula flowers in Crock-Pot and cover with oil. Cover Crock-Pot and set the temperature to low. Allow to infuse for 12 hours. Turn Crock-Pot off and infuse for 12 more hours, covered. Strain and discard plant matter. Heat the oil in the top of a double boiler with the beeswax. Stir until melted. Remove from heat. Stir until cooled and well blended. Pour into jar. Allow to cool completely and cover with a tight-fitting lid. If too thick for your liking, re-melt and add a little more oil. If too runny, add a little more beeswax.

Rose Moisturizer
2 large handfuls of fresh rose petals
1/4 cup apricot kernel oil
1 1/2 teaspoon beeswax
1 teaspoon wheat germ oil
15 drops rose geranium essential oil

Place rose petals in a wide-mouthed glass jar and cover with sweet almond oil. Bruise the petals with a spoon to start the maceration process. Seal the jar and place it in a sunny window for three weeks. Shake the mixture daily. Strain off the rose infused oil.
Heat the beeswax in the infused oil until melted. Add the wheat germ oil and the essential oil. Cool to room temperature. Pour the mixture into a dark a wide-mouthed jar and keep in a cool dry location. This will last two months at room temperature and four months if kept in the refrigerator.

Old Fashioned Rose Lotion
1/2 cup rose water
1/2 cup vegetable glycerin
20 drops vitamin E oil

Mix all ingredients together and store in dark glass bottles. Keep the lotion in a cool, dry cupboard.

Infused Rose Oil
Several handfuls of fresh rose petals
Enough sweet almond oil to cover

Place petals in a jar. Cover with oil. Put lid on tightly and shake well. Leave the mixture to steep in a warm room. Shake every day and remove blackened petals, replacing with fresh rose petals. Repeat until the scent is to your liking. Strain and keep in dark glass bottles in cool dry cupboard. The oil will keep for 6-12 months.

Uplifting Massage Oil
Fill a jar with rose geranium leaves and lavender buds. Cover with sweet almond oil. Cover tightly and steep in the sun for two weeks. Strain the liquid store in a dark glass bottle in a cool location away from the sun.

Relaxing Bath or Massage Oil
3/4 cup jojoba oil
1 teaspoon rose geranium essential oil

Pour into glass jar with a tight-fitting lid and shake well to blend. Keep jar in cool dark location. Use two teaspoons per bath.

Lavender and Peppermint Foot Lotion
3 tablespoons dried lavender flowers
2/3 cup distilled water
5 tablespoons glycerin
5 tablespoons witch hazel
6 drops peppermint essential oil

Place lavender and water in a saucepan. Bring to a boil. Cover and simmer 5 minutes. Cool and strain. Pour decoction into sterilized bottle or jar and add glycerin, witch hazel, and peppermint essential oil. Shake until well blended. Shake before each use. Use within two months.

Lavender Dusting Powder
1/4 cup arrowroot powder
1/4 cup cornstarch
3 tablespoons brown rice flour
6 drops lavender essential oil

Mix dry ingredients. Add essential oil. Mix well. Shelf life is one year.

Soothing Body Powder
2 tablespoons dried lavender
2 tablespoons dried calendula
1 tablespoon dried chamomile
1 tablespoon lemon balm
1/2 cup finely ground oatmeal
3/4 cup cornstarch
1/4 cup baking soda

Reduce first four ingredients to the consistency of a fine powder. Put in container with the other ingredients. Seal. Shake until well blended. Store in a shaker can in cool dark cupboard.

Chamomile Powder
1 cup arrowroot powder
1/2 cup baking soda
1 tablespoon dried chamomile, finely ground

Mix ingredients and place in powder decanter.

Lavender and Rose Dusting Powder
2 cups cornstarch
1 cup oats, finely ground
1 cup brown rice flour
3/4 cups powdered rose petals
1/2 cup baking soda
3 tablespoons powdered dry lavender buds
1 tablespoon powdered arrowroot
1/4 teaspoon rose geranium essential oil

Mix dry ingredients. Sprinkle essential oil over the powder mixture and mix well. Cover and allow it to sit for two weeks. Shake bottle daily. Transfer to shaker jars. This powder will last a year or more.

Chapter 7

Hands-on Skin Care

Sensitive Skin Characteristics

1. Develops rashes
2. Blushes easily
3. Overacts to extreme termperatures
4. Sunburns easily
5. Rosacea
6. Thread veins
7. Tends to be normal-to-dry or very dry

Avoid

1. Alcohol-based toners
2. Gritty facial scrubs
3. Herbal steams
4. Drying clay masks
5. Stimulating herbs
6. Alpha hydroxy and glycolic acids
7. Synthetic fragrance
8. Synthetic preservatives
9. Extremes of heat or cold
10. Terry wash cloths and coarse sponges
11. Tanning

Note: It is important to limit alcohol and tobacco use. Also, exercise is vital to your physical and mental health. Sweating cools the skin and eliminates waste. But, too much strenuous exercise can have adverse effects on people with sensitive skin. Remember the wise old saying, "Everything in moderation."

Application

Sensitive skin should not be overly stimulated, especially the face and décolleté area. Because these areas are often exposed to sun, wind, heat, and cold, they are often more sensitive than the arms, legs, and body. The skin on the elbows, hands, knees, and feet is tougher and often needs exfoliated to remove the build-up of dead skin cells so that new skin cells can generate and soft, healthy skin can be revealed.

Harsh scrubs are not recommended for sensitive skin, but a diluted scrub used as a polish can be administered with a gentle touch. For this process of gentle exfoliation, the eye area and areas affected by rosacea, acne, or couperose skin should be avoided as not to irritate delicate skin or exacerbate already irritated skin.

Sensitive skin is often dry, especially around the lips, nose, forehead, and the perimeter of the face, and can be gently exfoliated with a mild exfoliant mixture made of almond meal, finely ground oatmeal and powdered milk. It is imperative to avoid over-exfoliation. Always perform a thorough skin analysis first.

Prior to exfoliation, thoroughly cleanse the skin with a mild, creamy cleanser free of synthetics and stimulating essential oils. Lavender essential oil, mixed with a carrier oil, makes a good pre-cleanse, which will gently loosen debris on the skin's surface.

The pre-cleansing oil should be applied in a sweeping, side-to-side motion across the décolleté and up the neck. Move from the center and out, across the jaw line, around the mouth and nose, up the bridge of the nose, around the eyes and across the forehead.

For cleansing, a pure Castile liquid cleanser or a mild cream cleanser works best for sensitive skin. Again, apply from the décolleté up. Add a small amount of water to the palm of the hand and work the cleanser into the skin in circular motions. Use a soft cloth to remove the cleanser. Work gently from the forehead down.

Once the skin is thoroughly cleansed, it is important to use a gentle toner, which will remove any residue from the cleanser and restore the skin's natural pH balance. A good toner will also pull the moisturizer into the skin. Do not use alcohol-based toners on sensitive skin. The best natural gentle toners include rose water and witch hazel.

Sometimes, even they can be drying, so it is advisable to cut them with distilled water to make a half and half mixture that will not dry the skin out. A few drops of rose geranium oil or a little bit of vegetable glycerin will add emollient properties to smooth and pleasantly scent the skin.

Pat toners on with cotton squares or spritz on and gently work into the skin with a gentle rolling motion. Both a rose water and witch hazel spritzer can be used to set makeup, as a refresher, or as an after-bath mist to cool the skin.

Appropriate essential oils can be added for customization. For extremely dry skin, pure aloe vera gel or juice works well as a moisturizing and firming toner. It can be applied in the same manner as witch hazel or rose water toners. Toner helps to remove any residue left by cleansers, restores the pH balance, relaxes the pores so that they appear smaller, and pulls the moisturizer into the skin.

Now that the skin has been cleansed and the pH balance restored, a mild exfoliant can be used and worked into the skin with light pressure in a circular motion working from the décolleté to the forehead. It is very important to monitor the skin closely throughout the process to watch for irritation. Steam and steam towels should not be used when working with sensitive skin since it is prone to rosacea and couperous conditions (areas of redness with visibly broken capillaries). Extremes of heat should be avoided. It is important to keep sensitive skin calm.

Because stimulating massage is not an option for sensitive skin, pressure point is recommended at this point in the facial. Facial pressure point should always start on the forehead, at the hairline. Walk the hands down the face moving at the same time from the center outward. Each pressure point is activated first with a three-count pressure, three clockwise circular movements, three-count pressure, three circular movements counterclockwise, and finally, three-count pressure. Activate pressure points both right and left of the center of the face, simultaneously.

For sensitive skin, the mask process should be hydrating, soothing, and mildly drawing. Finely ground oatmeal, powdered milk, honey, and emollients such as shea butter and apricot kernel oil can be used as mask ingredients for sensitive skin. The main purpose of a sensitive skin facial is to thoroughly cleanse and calm the skin. Always avoid extremes of heat and cold. While the mask is setting, a scalp, hand and arm, or foot and leg massage can help in the calming and relaxation process. When we are relaxed, our skin is relaxed and more accepting of treatment.

Chapter 8

Would You Put That in Your Mouth?

We exercise our bodies and watch what we eat. But, when it comes to our skin, we'll just grab something off the shelves and smear it all over our bodies without even questioning what it contains.

Beauty does not come from a bottle. It is a direct result of eating a proper diet, getting daily exercise and adequate sleep, and by following an appropriate cleansing routine.

Healthy skin is a sign of good health. If your skin is dry and flaky, or oily and pimply, it can be a sign of internal or nutritional problems.

It is important to eat a healthy diet high in complex carbohydrates, low in fat, high in fiber, and a moderate amount of protein. Eat several servings of fresh and dried fruits, veggies, and whole grains. Also, nuts and seeds should be consumed daily. Try to stick to non-fat dairy products and limit yourself to three to four ounces of meat per day.

Contact dermatitis, which produces itchiness, redness, swelling, and mild fever, is the most common skin disorder. Fragrance can cause an immediate reaction. Weaker irritants may take up to ten days to trigger an allergic response. Lips, eyes, ears, neck, and hands are the most common sites for cosmetic allergies.

Synthetic fragrances can trigger asthma, detergents in shampoos can cause damage to eye tissue, and hair dye chemicals can cause bladder cancer and lymphoma.

It is important to know what is in the products you use every day and the best way to do that is to learn what to look for in a product ingredient label.

One good rule of thumb is, "If you wouldn't put it in your mouth . . . Don't put it on your skin." Your skin is your body's largest organ. Everything you put on it is absorbed into it. The toxic chemicals can be stored in fatty tissues or organs such as the liver, kidney, breasts, ovaries, and brain.

According to *The Green Beauty Guide*, by Julie Gabriel, scientists are finding phthalates (a component of plastic) in urine (Adibi et al., 2008), parabens, and antibacterial agents such as triclosan in breast tumor tissue (Darbre 2006) and the hormone-disrupting fragrant component xylene in human breast milk (Reiner et al., 2007).

The following list of synthetic ingredients is not comprehensive. For more information on harmful synthetic ingredients visit the Environmental Working Group's Skin Deep Cosmetics Database at www.ewg.org/skindeep.

1,4-dioxane

Very few, if any, skin care products list 1,4-dioxane as an ingredient, because it is a contaminant produced during manufacturing and therefore is not required to be listed as an ingredient.

1,4-dioxiane, a known cancer-causing agent, is found in up to 22 percent of the twenty-five thousand products on the market, and is most commonly found in products that create suds, like shampoo, liquid soap, and bubble bath. In addition to sodium laureth sulfate, other common ingredients that may be contaminated by 1,4-dioxane include (PEG) polyethylene glycol: oleth, myreth, and ceteareth.

Recent laboratory studies show that 1,4-dioxane is non-existent in products approved by the USDA National Organic Program.

Aluminum

Commonly found in deodorants, aluminum draws ions into the cells. When water flows in, the cells begin to swell, which prevents the secretion of sweat. Aluminum is a strong neurotoxin and contributes to both breast cancer and Alzheimer's disease.

Bronopol

One of the strongest lung and skin toxicants, 2-bromo-2-nitropropane-1,3-diol can contribute to the formation of cancer-causing nitrosamines, according to the FDA. It can also break down to produce formaldehyde. It is an endocrine disruptor and skin irritant.

DMDM-hydantoin

Contains formaldehyde.

Hydroquinone

Most often found in skin lighteners. It can also be found in facial and skin cleansers, facial moisturizer, and hair conditioners, listed as tocopherol acetate, or any ingredient with the root word "toco."

These chemicals decrease the production of melatonin pigments in the skin. By reducing melatonin, it increases exposure to UVA and UVB rays deep in the skin. The combination of UV exposure and carcinogens greatly increases the risk of developing cancer.

The Environmental Working Group's Skin Deep database, which compares cosmetic ingredients to more than fifty international toxics databases, identifies hydroquinone as a carcinogen, immunotoxicant and developmental and reproductive toxicant.

Imidazolidinyl Urea and Diazolidinyl Urea
Also known as Germall 115 and Germall 11, are a mixture of allantoin, urea, and formaldehyde, which are known skin irritants.

Iodopropynyl Butylcarbamate (IPBC)
A common wood preservative used in cosmetics, because of the iodine content, which may be absorbed into the bloodstream and affect the function of the thyroid gland because it contains Diethanolamine. It is also a gastrointestinal and liver toxicant and causes allergic contact dermatitis.

Lead
Possible human carcinogen and neurotoxin; skin and eye irritant.

Nitrosamines
A known contaminant found in nearly every kind of personal care product including mascara, concealer, conditioner, baby shampoo, pain relief salve and sunless tanning lotion.

Parabens
Parabens prevent the growth of microbes in cosmetic products. They can be absorbed through the skin, blood, and digestive system and have been found in biopsies from breast tumors at concentrations similar to those found in consumer products.

They are found in nearly all urine samples, on all socioeconomic levels, ethnic, and geographic backgrounds throughout the United States.

They are usually listed as ethylparaben, butylparaben, methylparaben, and propylparaben. Methylparaben and propylparaben can be found in more than ten thousand of the twenty-five thousand products in the Environmental Working Group's **Skin Deep** database.

Parabens have been linked to cancer, endocrine disruption, reproductive toxicity, immunotoxicity, neurotoxicity, and skin irritation. They adversely affect the hypothalamus, the ovaries, and the thyroid. Parabens mimic estrogen by binding to estrogen receptors on cells. They also increase the expression of genes usually regulated by estradiol.

Parabens have only been tested on short-term effects and can still be used in cosmetic products at levels of up to 25 percent of the finished product.

They are disguised on product labels as benzoic acid, isobutyl p-hydroxybenzoate, or p-methoxycarbonylphenol.

Phthalates
Often show up on labels as dialkyl, or alkyl aryl esters of 1, 2-benzenedicarboxylic acid in products such as shower curtains, rubber ducks, PVC furniture, clothes, sex toys, MP3 players, perfumes, and nail polishes.

Phthalates are linked to reproductive birth defects and other illnesses. The smell of a new car is nothing more than the smell of toxins emitting from a hot plastic car interior.

Constant exposure to phthalates increases the risk of developing cancer, diabetes, allergies, and infertility.
Caution: Pregnant women should not ride in a new car during the first trimester of pregnancy.

All synthetically scented products, including perfumes, contain phthalates in the form of di-n-butyl phthalate or DBP, commonly found in nail polish, di 2-ethylhexyl phthalate (DEHP), commonly found in perfumes, but most of the time they are hiding under the word "fragrance."

Phthalates have been linked to polycystic ovarian syndrome, infertility, and breast cancer. They can also cause damage to developing testes in males, which could result in low sperm count, sexual dysfunction, and hormonal imbalance.

They are also directly linked to abdominal obesity, breast cancer, and uterine cancer in women as well as insulin resistance and testicular cancer in men.

Propylene Glycol
Although it was banned from being used in cat food in 2001, propylene glycol can still be found in baby washes, bubble baths, deodorants, shampoos, hair dyes, and personal lubricants and has been deemed safe for use in foods, cosmetics, and medicines.

Ethylene Glycol
Commonly found in high doses in children's shampoos and baby washes, it is also used in antifreeze, deicing fluids, photographic developing solution, hydraulic brake fluid, and ink.

Diethylene Glycol
Is a known toxin and can be found in polyethylene glycol in very low doses.

Polyethylene Glycol (PEG)
Frequently used in "natural" cosmetics, laxatives, and syrupy medications. It is also used as a food preservative. It is a suspected endocrine disruptor; skin and eye irritant.

It should not be used on damaged skin. The most common reaction is contact dermatitis.

It aggravates acne and eczema, provokes skin irritation and sensitization in humans. Impurities found in PEG compounds include ethylene oxide, 1,4-dioxine, polycyclic aromatic compounds, and heavy metals including lead, iron, cobalt, nickel, cadmium, and arsenic.

Quaternium-15
Releases formaldehyde. Can cause skin and eye irritation. Linked to cancer.

A product is not green, natural, or organic if it contains petrochemicals such as mineral oil and silicone, sodium laureth, or lauryl sulfates or other sulfate-based detergents; propylene glycol, polyethylene glycol, and other ingredients made with PEGs or PGs; formaldehyde and paraben, synthetic dyes and colorants, or artificial fragrance.

Note: Natural skin care products can also trigger sensitivity, but it is easily corrected by removing or replacing the offending ingredient, just as you would with food allergies. First starting out, use products with only a few ingredients and make adjustments when needed depending on stress level, the seasons, and your age. Your skin will adapt. Just know that when your skin is healthy, it will be able to heal itself. Always pay attention to what your skin is trying to tell you.

Bibliography

Balch, Phyllis A., CNC, *Prescription for Nutritional Healing, Fourth Edition:A Practical A-Z Reference to Drug-Free Remedies Using Vitamins, Minerals, Herbs & Food Supplements,* New York, New York, Penguin Group, 2006.

Breedlove, Greta, *The Herbal Home Spa: Naturally Refreshing Wraps, Rubs, Lotions, Masks, Oils and Scrubs,* Pownal, Vermont, Storey Books, 1998.

Bremness, Lesley, *The Complete Book of Herbs: A practical guide to growing & using herbs,* New York, New York, Penguin Books, 1994.

Chevalier, Andrew, *Herbal Remedies,* New York, New York, DK Publishing, 2007.

Cox, Lauren w/Janice Cox, *Ecobeauty: Scrubs, Rubs, Masks and Bath Bombs for You and Your Friends,* New York, New York, Ten Speed Press, 2009.

Fairley, Josephine, *The Ultimate Natural Beauty Book: 100 organic beauty products to make and use easily at home,* New York, New York, Universe Publishing, 2004.

Freeman, Sally, *Everywoman's Guide to Ageless Natural Beauty,* Garden City, New York, Bookspan, 2000.

Gabriel, Julie, *The Green Beauty Guide: Your Essential Resource to Organic and Natural Skin Care, Hair Care, Makeup, and Fragrance,* Deerfield Beach, Florida, Health Communications, Inc., 2008.

Grieve, Mrs. M., *A Modern Herbal, The Medicinal, Culinary, Cosmetic and Economic Properties, Cultivation and Folk-Lore of Herbs, Grasses, Fungi Shrubs & Trees with Their Modern Scientific Uses, Volumes I & II,* New York, New York, Dover Publishers, 1971.

Griggs, Barbara, *The Green Witch Herbal: Restoring Nature's Magic in Home, Health & Beauty Care,* Rochester, Vermont, Healing Arts Press, 1994.

Garrett, Ginger. *Beauty Secrets of the Bible,* Nashville, Tennessee, Thomas Nelson, Inc., 2007.

Mabey, Richard, *The New Age Herbalist: How to use herbs for healing, nutrition, body care, and relaxation,* New York, London, Tornonto, Sydney, Simon & Schuster Inc., 1988.

Malkan, Stacy, *Not Just a Pretty Face: The Ugly Side of the Beauty Industry,* Gabriola Island, BC, Canada, New Society Publishers, 2007.

Tourles, Stephanie, *The Herbal Body Book: A Natural Approach to Healthier Hair, Skin and Nails,* Pownal, Vermont, Storey Publishing, 1994.

Index